The Chocolate Diet Book

Sally Ann Voak

JOHN BLAKE

Published by Blake Publishing Ltd,
3 Bramber Court, 2 Bramber Road, London W14 9PB, England

ISBN 1 85782 437 7

British Library Cataloguing-in-Publication Data:
A catalogue record for this book is available from
the British Library.

Typeset by Jon Davies

Printed in Great Britain by CPD, Wales

1 3 5 7 9 10 8 6 4 2

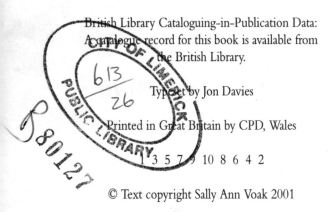

Papers used by John Blake Ltd are natural, recyclable products
made from wood grown in sustainable forests. The manufacturing
processes conform to the environmental regulations of the country
of origin.

Contents

1

What is a Chocaholic?

The word 'chocoholic' trips smoothly off the tongue ... just like the creamy peppermint filling of a dark, crunchy after-dinner mint. But what does the term really mean?

Chocoholism is often mentioned in advertisements to promote confectionery and is used glibly by reed-thin models who might eat a bar of chocolate once a week. People take alcoholism seriously but chocoholism is often just an amusing term to describe weak-willed people who can't resist the occasional 'pig-out' on chocolate. If this is true, why are so many people unable to control their insatiable craving for it and why do they long to reduce their chocolate intake?

Frankly, for millions of serious chocolate addicts, there is nothing amusing about chocoholism. Just like the addiction to any drug (and chocolate could almost be described as a 'drug' for it contains chemicals which can affect the body and brain), chocolate addiction takes over your life. The few moments of pleasure you enjoy as you eat that bagful of chocolate truffles, milky bar or tube of chocolate-covered caramels are quickly forgotten as you pay the awful price – guilt, self-disgust and an overwhelming desire for another 'fix'. Chocolate can become as irresistible as sex, as habit-forming as smoking, and as difficult to give up as both.

What's more, eating too much chocolate makes most addicts put on weight. Chocolate is one of the most fattening 'treats' ever invented because it contains sugar and fat and is high in calories. Eating too much of it has a disturbing effect on the body's blood sugar levels, so cutting down or giving up becomes very diffcult indeed. So anyone with a weight problem who is a chocoholic will find it twice as difficult if they try to shed their excess pounds. It is a bit like being on a roller-coaster ride — you are 'high' one minute, 'low' the next and hungry all the time.

In this book, I have set out to prove that it is possible to break that vicious circle and lose weight. What's more, you can even learn to eat chocolate in moderation and enjoy every mouthful.

How to Tell If You Are a Chocaholic

As you have bought this book, there is a very strong chance that you are a chocoholic. Perhaps seeing it on the bookstall made you finally admit to yourself that you do have a problem. Here is a very simple quiz to help you find out for sure. Just answer 'Yes' or 'No' to the 20 questions below, then check your score.

1. Are you eating chocolate while you are doing this quiz?

Yes / ~~No~~

2. Did you buy *The Chocolate Diet Book* because you are worried about your chocolate cravings?

~~Yes~~ / No

3. Did your mum or dad give you chocolate as a reward or comforting treat when you were a child?

Yes / ~~No~~

4. Have you ever hidden a secret hoard of chocolate in a drawer, cupboard, under the bed or in some other hideaway?

Yes / ~~No~~

5. Do you frequently buy chocolate when you set out to shop for other things — i.e. at the supermarket check-out or garage?

~~Yes~~ / No

6. Have you ever sneaked into the loo at work or at home for a chocolate 'fix'?

Yes / ~~No~~

7. Does your closest relative know how much chocolate you eat?

~~Yes~~ / ~~No~~

8. Do you eat chocolate after a row with your partner?

~~Yes~~ / ~~No~~

9. Do you always choose the chocolate gateau or mousse on restaurant dessert trolleys?

Yes / ~~No~~

10. Do you ever eat more than one bar of chocolate or a whole box of chocolates or packet of biscuits at one sitting?

Yes / No

11. Would you rather eat something chocolate than a proper meal?

Yes / No

12. Do you crave chocolate when you see it advertised on television or in magazines?

Yes / No

13. Does eating chocolate make you feel more loved and loving?

Yes / No

14. Do all your friends buy you chocolates because they know how much you adore them?

Yes / No

15. Have you ever started a crash diet before Christmas or Easter so you can eat more chocolate over the holiday?

Yes / No

16. Does eating chocolate seem to give you extra energy?

Yes / No

17. Do you normally eat chocolate alone rather than with other people?

Yes / No

18. Do you think your consumption of chocolate is responsible for your weight problems?

Yes / No

19. Have you tried to control your lust for chocolate and failed?

 Yes / No

20. Imagine you are marooned on a desert island with just a grass skirt, a Bounty Bar and some chocolate coins. The natives have offered you a boat in return for your chocs. Would you trade?

Yes / No

How Did You Score?

Give yourself one point for every 'Yes' answer, with the exception of question 7. (Give yourself a point for answering 'No' to that question.

Less than 5 points? You are a serious chocolate lover who is not yet a chocoholic. However, you are already treading on dangerous ground. For a start, you have yet to learn how to control your consumption of chocolate properly. Do you eat it because you like it, or in response to pressure, or because you crave chocolate for its comfort value? Reading this book will help you find out. If you have a weight problem, you can certainly try one of the diet plans in Chapter Six.

Between 5 and 15 points? Yes, you are a chocoholic. You must sort out your problems now — before it becomes a dangerous addiction. Chocolate is beginning to take over your life, so now is the time to break this pattern for good. Your chocoholism is making you sneaky, moody, unhappy and fatter than you should be. The good news is that you have already taken the first step towards beating it. Well done!

Over 15 points? Wow! You are seriously addicted to chocolate. Thank goodness you bought this book. Read it carefully and follow all our advice. There is a list of counsellors and groups on page 235, who will be able to give you extra help. Please don't be nervous about seeking it. Your chocoholism is very serious indeed. Do write to me at the address on page 236, and let me know how you get on with the diet.

What's in Chocolate?

The cocoa bean contains 50 per cent fat, 20–25 per cent carbohydrate, 5 per cent water, 1.5 per cent theobromine, tyramine and 3.5 per cent minerals and vitamins. These include potassium, calcium, iron, magnesium, sodium, phospherous, Vitamin A, thiamine, Riboflavin and niacin.

It also contains a powerful chemical called phenylethylamine, which is found in the human brain. This is a natural amphetamine which is activated when we are in love giving that wonderful 'out of this world' feeling of euphoria.

When cocoa is made into chocolate, a lot of sugar is added — around two-fifths of its weight. Milk chocolate contains even more sugar, plus milk solids. When this sugar gets into your bloodstream it gives you an instant 'high'. This triggers the pancreas into releasing large amounts of insulin to deal with the rise in blood sugar. Unfortunately, ten minutes or so later, your blood sugar level drops dramatically, producing a 'low' and a craving for more.

Chocolate also contains a small amount of caffeine. Although there is far more in a cup of tea or coffee, if you have a chocolate binge you are likely to experience some effects from the caffeine such as flushed cheeks and palpitations.

Ten Reasons Why Chocolate Makes You Fat

1. Chocolate is the ultimate comfort food. Parents offer it to their children to cheer them up. So, later on we offer it to ourselves when things go wrong. That's why you rush into a sweetshop for a Snickers or a Mars bar when you've had a row with the boss. That's also the reason why you dig into the choccy biscuit tin when you're watching a weepie movie on TV, or have to reprimand your kids for bad behaviour.

2. It is mega-high in calories. If lettuce was as comforting and delicious as chocolate, very few people

would have a weight problem. But lettuce contains only 3 calories an ounce, whereas even just a small (50g) bar of dark chocolate will 'cost' about 250 calories. Since most women put on weight on more than 2000 calories daily, chocolate is dangerous. You only need a couple of bars daily, plus your normal diet, to push your weight up ... and up!

3. Chocs are not filling. Your body feels cheated when you replace a proper, balanced meal with chocolate. So, it responds by craving more! Chocolate contains sugar and fat. Unfortunately, unless it is the nutty kind, it contains no fibre, which is the stuff that makes your tummy feel full and send 'satisfied' messages to your brain. So, unless you are physically sick, it's hard to tell when you have had enough.

4. You can eat chocolate anywhere. It is socially acceptable to stuff your face with chocolate in the street, at a party, at your desk, on a train. It is less messy to munch a Crunchie bar than a sandwich while you wait for a bus. It is easier to stash away a pack of

m&ms than a tub of healthy cottage cheese in your handbag.

5. It is so available! You cannot leave the safety of your own home without being assailed by chocolates — they're shouting 'buy me, eat me' wherever you go — in the garage, in the supermarket, in vending machines, you name it. It's unfair!

6. Chocolate gives you a 'high' as I explained above. This happens when the chemicals, theobromine and tyramine, which chocolate contains are combined with refined sugar. But this is followed by a fall in your blood sugar which makes you immediately crave another 'fix', and this can rapidly become a binge. This effect is intensified if you combine chocolate with caffeine, so cola and coffee drinkers are even more likely to binge.

7. Chocolate can be a substitute for sex. Sounds far-fetched? In fact, chocolate contains a chemical called phenylethylamine which the brain produces when we

are in love. This explains why slimmers who have troubled love lives often get choccy cravings. If your weight problems are related to your sex life (and they often are), eating chocolate will make things worse.

8. Advertisements promote chocolate as an exciting treat. A beautiful girl, dressed only in hideously expensive underwear, sits at a window. Sensuously, she bites into a phallic-shaped bar of chocolate and gazes out into the mist. She is obviously waiting for a handsome bloke to arrive and the chocolate is helping her get into a sexy mood ... Cor! If you are trying to cope with two difficult kids, tidy up last night's mess, answer the telephone and do the ironing all at the same time, the idea of a bar of chocolate becomes very appealing indeed. Two bars would be even nicer ... and so it goes on!

9. Premenstrual food cravings often include chocolate. Just when women are particularly vulnerable, before their monthly period, chocs appear most attractive. With hormones going haywire, causing fluid retention

and mood swings, chocolate seems like a soothing drug. Sadly, it just makes things worse.

10. There are no taboos about eating chocolate. Although you may be ashamed of your chocolate addiction, society doesn't frown on you for eating it. If you sat in the pub drinking gin all day, people would talk. But sitting at home stuffing Mars bars is OK. It isn't though, is it?

2

Chocolate and History

When you consider chocolate's sensual taste and exotic background it isn't surprising that it is considered such a treat. For centuries, only the very rich could afford it and most of them couldn't eat — or drink — enough to have to worry about its fattening powers. These days, it is available to everyone and costs relatively little compared with other luxury foods.

The ancient Aztecs were the very first chocoholics. They grew the first cacao trees in the

Amazon basin in about AD600, and preferred to grind the beans, mix them with chilli powder and serve the resulting brew topped up with water as a frothy drink called Chocolatl. In 1519, the famous Aztec Emperor Moctezuma (Montezuma) entertained the Spanish explorer Hernando Cortés with a banquet which included 50 large jugs of Chocolatl, served up in pure gold cups. When Cortés returned to Spain (after killing poor Moctezuma and conquering Mexico), he took some cocoa beans with him.

At first, the Spanish were not very impressed by the taste of Chocolate prepared the Aztec way. It gave them severe tummy ache (known later as Montezuma's Revenge!) and was very bitter and unpalatable. However, when sugar and vanilla beans were also brought back from the New World, they were added to the ground-up cocoa beans to make a more palatable drink which they found very acceptable.

For about 100 years, the Spanish had a monopoly of the chocolate trade. Meanwhile, cocoa beans were used as currency in Central America, which meant that most people could not afford to drink chocolate.

Ten beans would buy you a rabbit, and a woman for the night, and for a mere 100 beans you could purchase a reasonably fit slave, so choccy 'money' was obviously far too precious to waste.

At the beginning of the fifteenth century, chocolate was introduced in Italy and France and became highly fashionable. Princess Maria-Thérèse of Spain adored it so much that she persuaded her husband, King Louis XIV of France, to try it. He became hooked too and the royal couple had a special 'chocolate-making' maid to prepare it.

Although chocolate was thought to have restorative powers, it must have caused quite a few spreading waistlines among the super rich, for it was very high indeed in fat. The cocoa bean is about 50 per cent fat, so when the drink was made, this would rise to the surface. Some could be spooned off but the majority remained. When the first chocolate house opened in London in 1657, the drink was so fatty that flour, oatmeal or arrowroot was added to counteract this. But, in 1828, a Dutchman named Coenraad Van Houten developed a hydraulic press which removed most of the cocoa butter, leaving behind cocoa powder.

This invention paved the way for Englishmen John Cadbury and Joseph Fry to start producing chocolate bars by blending the ground-up beans with sugar and additional cocoa butter. From the mid-1860s onwards, eating chocolate became more and more popular, and the types of chocolate available became more elaborate. Fancy chocolate assortments began to be sold in beautiful containers, including velvet-covered mirrored caskets and hand-painted boxes. The French and Swiss became masters of the exotic chocolate gift, but it was not too long before the English manufacturers caught up and they in turn were closely followed by the Americans.

It is interesting that many of the first great chocolate manufacturers were also great philanthropists too. Joseph Fry, Henry Rowntree and John Cadbury were all Quakers, attracted to chocolate because, like tea and coffee, it is non-alcoholic. They cared for their workers, providing free medical check-ups, uniforms and even exercise sessions. In France, chocolatier Jean

Menier built the first 'chocolate village' for his workers, and, in 1879, George and Richard Cadbury, sons of John, followed suit with the famous village of Bournville, near Birmingham. Today, their newest plant can wrap 15,000 bars of chocolate every hour. In America, Milton Hershey built a model town called Hersheyville, where the famous Hershey bar was developed as a high-energy food for soldiers during World War II.

Chocolate and Easter

The craze for eating chocolate Easter eggs made chocolate production become an even bigger money-making industry. Eggs had always been associated with Easter; they are a symbol of fertility, which ties in naturally with the festival of Spring. When the church in Europe adopted the pagan festival of Easter (or Eostre), some regarded eggs as the symbol of the stone being rolled away from Jesus's tomb. Before chocolate, eggs were either painted real ones, or made from anything from precious stones to cardboard.

The French and German chocolate-makers attempted the first chocolate eggs, painstakingly painting individual moulds with paste chocolate. The first British eggs were made in 1875, when Cadbury found a method of making chocolate flow into the moulds. Now, the basic shell shape (which is usually the least calorific part of the egg as it is very thin) is often a container for everything from toys to more choc-bars.

For chocoholics, the Easter festival is nothing short of a fat-making nightmare. Lured into supermarkets and sweetshops by the sight of dozens of beautiful, delicious eggs, chocoholics can hardly be expected to resist them. Sitting innocently on the shelf, those eggs give out a powerful combination of sex, fertility, and irresistible chemical power. No wonder we are almost compelled to buy them. The best way to deal with this temptation is to be aware of the calorie content of the chocolates and eggs you buy, and to go for the lower-calorie sort, and be very determined to eat just one egg, instead of a dozen. The popular Cadbury's Creme Egg is always a good choice, as it contains just 175 calories and is very satisfying in every way!

Sex, Lust and Choc-Erotica

So, is chocolate an aphrodisiac? The early choc-lovers certainly thought so. After all, they had never tried anything remotely like it before. It came from an exotic country, was expensive, sensual-tasting, and had the added advantage of making you feel loved and loving. (Of course, they did not know about phenylethylamine, the chemical that fools the brain into making chocolate-eaters think they are in love, but that did not stop them from experiencing those loving urges!)

They had also heard the legends about the incredible potency of chocolate as a love-making potion: Moctezuma apparently drank vast quantities of it before visiting his wives and instructed his cocoa planters to have sexual intercourse on top of the young growing plants to speed up their growth. Wow! Casanova was also convinced about the aphrodisiac powers of chocolate. He thought that giving his conquests a draught of hot chocolate was a better bet than plying them with champagne which, although it got them in the mood for love, left them feeling too tired and emotional for vigorous action. Today, chocolates are often the very first gift presented to a woman by a new lover or by an old one who fears that love has gone off the boil. Subconsciously, he is hoping that they will inflame his beloved to heights of passion. It may work, but unfortunately too many gifts like that could make his beloved too fat to fondle! The idea of being given a box of chocs is so delicious that very few women can refuse the offer. Even if your man is unlikely to land by helicopter, scale a cliff, then swim through a swamp to bring you your box of Milk Tray, his heart is obviously in the right place if he bothers to buy one at all. Taking chocolate, or chocolates, to bed when you are lonely is, therefore, a very logical thing for a woman to do, for the comfort and 'lift' of the chocs seems like the perfect substitute for a man. Again, this can be dangerous, as going to bed with a man will help you burn off calories, whereas spending too many nights in bed with only chocolate for company will certainly make you put on pounds.

Women have traditionally used chocolate to perk up their men, too. The famous French courtier Madame du Barry apparently gave it to her lovers if they were feeling a bit droopy. The restorative powers of chocolate were thought to be so effective that a seventeenth-century English gentleman would pop into a chocolate house to sip a large tot before visiting his mistress. Or the mistress would have a cup of hot chocolate ready in the bedchamber to get the poor chap in the mood. Think about that next time you make your partner a steaming cup of chocolate at the end of a busy day. Monks were banned from drinking it in case their ardours got out of hand, and an article written in *The Spectator* in May 1712 warned readers about 'meddling with chocolates, novels and the like, which I look upon as very dangerous'.

Chocs That Shook

Once the manufacturers had discovered how to make chocolate flow into moulds its production became more sophisticated. Eggs were the first moulded chocolate novelties, but they were followed by a flood of unusual, and sometimes very risque, choccy gifts, particularly from the naughty French chocolatiers. Phallic-shaped chocs, chocolate breasts and bottoms could be obtained 'under the counter', while the normal business of selling eggs, bunnies and fondant-filled chocolates was carried on upstairs. Although all this naughtiness stopped during the war years and the austere 1950s, it came back with a bang in the sexy seventies when phallic chocs were sold at the popular sex shops along with other aids to rapturous love-making. Choc erotica is certainly thriving well in the naughty nineties. Rude chocs can now be bought openly in gift shops and are a big hit at Christmas time. One of the best sellers last year was a 'saucy stocking' containing two breasts, two bottoms and a penis. According to the London-based company who make this saucy item, it was bought mainly by women as a gift for their husbands. Madame du Barry obviously had the right idea.

My conclusion is that, in small doses, chocolate is definitely an aphrodisiac. A delicious nibble, tasted when you are in the right mood, with the right person, could turn you on to thoughts of love with all the accompanying physical feelings ... and very nice, too. The problems start when chocolate is eaten in large quantities, as a love substitute. That is when weight problems inevitably follow — which may make you feel depressed, unlovely, and unloving. A case in point is famous chocoholic and television personality, Nina Myscow, who says, 'When I lived alone, I frequently woke up in the night with the most awful chocolate cravings. Once, I even drove to an all-night supermarket just to buy a chocolate doughnut ... and then ate it before it defrosted! Now, I live with my boyfriend and I still occasionally eat chocolate in bed. These days, though, a little nibble is perfectly satisfying!'

Ten Hard-to-Follow Facts about Chocs

1. If all the Crunchies sold in a year were placed end to end, they would stretch from Birmingham to Bangkok and back.

2. If all the Creme Eggs made by Cadbury were stacked one on top of each other, the pile of chocs would be ten times higher than Mount Everest.

3. You could fill 60 double-decker buses with a year's production of Double Deckers.

4. Forty Kit Kats are consumed in the UK every second.

5. The amount of milk used in a year's production of Dairy Milk would fill 14 Olympic-size swimming pools.

6. If all the Wispa bars sold were laid end to end, they would stretch 3.15 times around the world.

7. The money spent on chocs and sweets in half-an-hour would pay for all the tickets to a Madonna concert.

8. The weight of chocolate sold each year in the UK is equivalent to the combined weight of 3,000 blue whales.

9. As a nation, we spend about £5 billion a year feeding our chocolate habit.

10. In the UK, we eat an average of 11kg of chocolate per person per year. However, the world's top consumers of chocolates are the Swiss, closely followed by the Norwegians, then the Belgians, Dutch and Germans.

Choccy Nutrient Guide

50 gram bar of	Plain	Milk	White
Calories	255	260	265
Fat (g)	14	15	15
Calcium (mg)	17	110	135
Iron (mg)	2.2	0.7	Trace
Magnesium (mg)	45	25	13

3

Reward, Comfort and Guilt

*H*ave you ever felt very low and miserable and longed for the comforting arms of your partner or mum, then eaten some chocolate instead? Most people have done exactly the same thing. In fact, there are very powerful reasons why this emotional response to chocolate occurs.

Our love of sweet foods, including chocolate, is strongly associated with childhood and mother love. The very first food a baby tastes is milk, which, like chocolate, has a high fat content. As it grows and tries different foods, a child will naturally go for those with the obvious kind of taste — strong things like tomato ketchup, sweets and chocolate. It is only later on, during adolescence, that our taste-buds develop to appreciate more subtle and sophisticated food and drink.

We become so sensitive to smells as well as tastes that we can differentiate between very similar tastes to an amazing degree. It is nature's way of helping us to 'tune in' to the wide variety of nutrients we need in our diet, and to learn the subtleties of sexuality — the smells and tastes of love. That is why we generally feel a bit childish when we pour a big dollop of tomato sauce on our sausages, or dive into a bag of m&ms. That childish feeling is also comforting because most of us naturally associate good things with that period of our lives — things such as security, warmth, and love. If our parents habitually rewarded us with sweets for good behaviour or gave us sweet foods when we were upset, then that feeling becomes even stronger.

Psychologist Jane Firbank says, 'People don't realise how much we are governed by these primitive feelings. Did you know, for instance, that the reason we take chocolates to people in hospital is because they have returned to a childlike, helpless state and therefore we feel they should be treated like children? This sounds very condescending, but is in fact flattering because we are offering them love, comfort and nurturing along with the chocs!'

Even the man who brings his girlfriend a box of chocolates is giving her motherly messages as well as sexual ones. 'In effect, he is saying, "I will take care of you,"' says Jane. 'He is able to do this without diminishing his own masculinity in any way, simply by giving the chocolates.'

Jewish mothers are renowned for thrusting food at their children as a love-offering but any mother will spend a lot of time nurturing her child with lovingly prepared food. The problems start when a mother forces her child to eat up chocolate puddings instead of chicken soup!

Jane says, 'If taken to extremes, this can be quite a dangerous thing. The mother is almost saying, "eat my food or you reject me". The child's response will probably be to eat up and shut up, but in later life, he or she may be strongly affected by this. A very dominant mum can push an entire family into chocoholism.'

So, what can a chocoholic do about this? Firstly, recognise that these are all very common problems, so you are not the only one who is likely to 'pig-out' as soon as things go wrong. Secondly, if you are overweight, it makes sense to get into better shape, using this book to help. Once you feel better about yourself, get out and about more, enjoy sports and generally have a good time, there will be fewer opportunities for you to become depressed and have to resort to those 'childish longings'! Following is a list of everyday situations which often trigger a choc attack, with some suggestions of alternative methods of dealing with them. Try them.

Swaps for Chocs

You don't have to deal with every tricky situation in your life by eating something sweet. But, if you have been conditioned by your parents to deal with 'hurt' by putting chocs into your mouth, it is very hard to kick the habit. You can do it — practice makes perfect.

Here's a guide to ten familiar daily problems and your probable choccy response together with some alternative suggestions.

Time   7am

Problem You've overslept — again. Your partner is unsympathetic and there is no time for breakfast.

Choc Response You buy a tube of chocolate caramels at the paper shop and eat them on the bus or train, kidding yourself that you need the instant energy.

Non-Choc Solution Make yourself a healthy salad sandwich the night before, wrap it in foil, and stick it in the fridge. You can eat that on the way to work, instead of the chocs.

Time   11am

Problem Your boss has just summoned you to his office for being late. You feel fed up and bored stiff with your work. The office trolley has just arrived on your floor.

Choc Response Your eyes alight on the Mars Bars on the trolley, and you buy two — wolfing them down so quickly that you feel queasy.

Non-Choc Solution Take a deep breath, apologise to the boss, and make a list of ways you can improve production in your section or jot down some ideas for a new project. Get stuck into your work so you don't even notice when the trolley comes around.

Time   1pm

Problem Your partner has just telephoned to cancel your lunch-date together because of pressure of work. You are disappointed and wonder if he or she is telling the truth.

Choc Response You go to the canteen and indulge in a massive lunch of burgers and chips with a bar of fruit and nut chocolate for dessert.

Non-Choc Solution Exercise is the best way to let off

steam. Go for a brisk walk in the park first, then have that canteen lunch. Chances are you'll pick a more balanced meal.

Time   4pm

Problem You suddenly remember that you have promised to give a talk to the Parents' Association at your child's school tonight. Sheer terror strikes — you haven't prepared a thing!

Choc Response You dig deep in your desk or locker and find a few of the chocolate biscuits you keep there. You gobble them up.

Non-Choc Solution Take deep breaths to help you relax. You know your subject and have bags of time to write a few ideas down on the journey home, so there's no need to panic.

Time   6pm

Problem Your partner is in a foul mood (work was hectic today) and starts up an old row about the state of the family's finances in general, and your extravagance in particular.

Choc Response You lock yourself in the loo with a stiff gin and a Mars Bar until the tirade is over.

Non-Choc Solution Put on a soothing tape or CD, sit down with your partner and plan the week's budget together.

Time   9pm

Problem Your talk has gone well but now you are landed with a group of boring parents moaning about fund-raising. They are getting on your nerves and you feel yourself being drawn towards the chocolate swiss roll on the refreshment table.

Choc Response You take three slices and wolf them down with a cup of coffee.

Non-Choc Solution Excuse yourself, politely, from the parents, make your excuses and go home — you have done your bit!

Time   10pm

Problem While you were out, your mother has phoned to ask why you forgot her birthday, yet again. She wants you to ring back as soon as you get home ...

Choc Response You know there is a Black Forest gateau in the fridge, so you cut a slice and eat it rapidly. Then, you ring your mum and grovel.

Non-Choc Solution You plan to send your mum flowers in the morning. You put on the anwering machine and watch the News on TV while you sip a soothing cup of tea.

Time   10.30pm

Problem You are feeling sexy, your partner is not and won't even give you a cuddle.

Choc response You creep downstairs for another slice of gateau and suffer from indigestion all night long. Result: neither of you get a wink of sleep.

Non-Choc Solution You tickle your partner's feet and tell them a silly, sexy joke. Laughter is the best aphrodisiac of the lot and less fattening than chocolate!

Why You Feel Guilty When You Don't Share Chocs

Why is it that eating a whole box of chocs alone is such a guilt-making experience? Have you ever watched one of those Natural History programmes on TV, where a whole colony of monkeys is studied in detail? Next time, watch out for the bit where they look at the way monkeys eat. Notice how, in normal feeding, the monkey is happy to find his own food and tuck into it, but when he finds something really special like a tree with some particularly tasty fruit, he shares it with the whole group. Well, we humans feel the same way.

When we are eating normal, everyday food (e.g. tucking into a bowl of cornflakes, or eating lunch in the canteen) there is absolutely no question of sharing our meal. In fact, our family or workmates would be rather taken aback if we did offer them a spoonful of cereal or a second-hand brussels sprout. But, 'luxury' foods like chocolate are very different. Instinctively, we feel that these foods must be shared out and we feel like the biggest meanie in the world if we eat them alone. That's why you feel so furious with yourself if you eat up a whole boxful of chocs. You may even lie about it to your family, using excuses like 'the dog had them', or 'I threw them away by mistake.'

Why You Can't Resist Chocolate Puddings

Imagine that you have been out with friends for a fantastic meal and decided to forget your diet for once. You started with a few drinks and nibbles, then had a substantial starter which was a meal in itself — a huge prawn cocktail, pasta dish, or fat-loaded pâté. Then, along comes the main course — steak, onion rings, chips, peas, plus a side-salad washed down with a few glasses of wine. You feel absolutely stuffed and decide not to have any pud.

Suddenly, the waiter wheels the sweet trolley up to your table, and you get a whiff of chocolate gateau.

Amazingly, your brain is suddenly telling you that your tummy is empty and you need some chocolate giteau, even though you most certainly don't. You succumb, and tuck into a huge slice.

Why did you do it? Blame nature! We are 'programmed' to eat a variety of foods in order to obtain the many different nutrients we need to keep our bodies ticking over. So, when a powerful new food, smelling and looking absolutely luscious, is presented to us after a meal, we can still find room for it. In effect, we are 'stocking up' with the luxury food in case we don't get offered any more for a long time. This is obviously nonsense, since we are very likely to have some more chocs the following day, but our primitive urges are very powerful indeed.

You can beat this, and similar potentially dangerous encounters with chocolate, by with some 'mind over body' exercises. Try these:

1. Before going out for a meal, sit down quietly and imagine yourself eating it. Make sure you have a clear picture in your mind of what will happen after

your main course. Picture yourself selecting the fresh fruit salad from the trolley. Keep that image tucked away for later on. You can do it!

2. Before you go to a supermarket, write a list of everything you need. Now picture yourself at the check-out. You walk past the sweet and chocolate counter and you do not put anything in your trolley.

3. Before you go into a fast-food restaurant, imagine yourself choosing a fairly sensible meal of burger, bun and fruit juice. After this meal you are feeling very full and satisfied, and do not want a chocolate shake or slice of gateau. In your imagination, you can see yourself getting up from the table and leaving the restaurant without succumbing to temptation.

4. Before you go to a friend's home for dinner, have a clear idea in your mind about the food you will be eating. Try to 'see' yourself sitting at the table, eating a good meal, but refusing the chocolate after-

dinner mints because you are just too full up to eat them. Go so far as to practise saying to your hostess, 'No thank you. The rest of the meal was so filling and delicious that I just haven't room for anything else.'

4

Overweight Chocaholics — The Big Six

As you will have learned by reading the first few chapters of this book, there are plenty of good reasons why people become hooked on chocolate. In fact, it's amazing that more people haven't succumbed to the 'disease', particularly in the United Kingdom, where £2.4 billion worth of chocolate is consumed annually. That is about £100 a second, and enough to buy 5,000 Rolls-Royces, 60 Jumbo jets, or 500 Michael Owens!

This figure is increasing by nearly 3 per cent per

annum. Today, we eat over 200 million Cadbury's Creme Eggs every year and enough Dairy Milk to cover all the pitches in the football league. If you've got a taste for this kind of statistic, recheck the list on page 28 when you feel a severe case of choccy cravings coming over you — the images they conjure up could help put you off. (If they don't, you certainly do need this book!)

Since the calories supplied by 25g of milk or plain chocolate is approximately 150, it is not surprising that many (although not all) chocoholics have weight problems. Although a mere 150 calories might not sound much, when you consider that the weight of a typical chocolate bar (such as a Galaxy) would be around 85g, it means that the total calories consumed in a whole bar would be over 400. A chronic chocoholic would have no trouble at all in putting away over 1000 calories of chocolate daily. If he or she is in a sedentary job and eats a fairly normal diet as well as the chocolate, that extra 1000 calories daily could result in a gradual weight-gain of around 2lb weekly.

At this point let me say that, in my 30 years' experience of working with slimmers, calories do count. Yes, I know that some lucky people can burn energy more quickly than others but the simple fact remains that if you consume fewer calories than you expend you will lose weight. Sorry, folks, it's painful but true. So, never trust a diet that says you can eat as much as you like of foods other than those that are so low in calories (e.g. green vegetables and salads) that you'd have to eat a ton to put on a pound. Certainly never trust a diet that says you can eat anything you like — even for just an hour or so a day. A determined chocoholic could easily stuff 3,000 calories worth of chocs in that time without pain (until later!).

A calorie is a unit of energy: the amount that, if converted into heat, would raise the temperature of 1 gram of water by 1 degree Centigrade. This is a very small unit indeed, so when scientists are measuring food intake, they use a unit that is a thousand times larger, called a kilocalorie (kcal for short). However, most slimming writers, including me, don't bother with the kilo prefix. All you really need to know is that the average woman in a sedentary job uses around 2,000 calories each day, and the average man will use something between 2,500 and 3,000 daily.

Some foods are more calorie intensive than others (i.e. they pack a whole lot of calories into a very small mouthful), particularly those high in fat-like cheese (116 calories for just a 28g chunk of Cheddar) or butter (210 calories per 25g). Sweet foods are calorie-intensive too. 25g of white, granulated sugar contains 112 calories, and even a level teaspoon can set you back 20 calories. Chocolate is high in fat and sugar, so it is one of the most calorie-intensive foods you can consume. When I call it a 'food', I mean just that because both fat and sugar are nutrients — although we should eat less of them. Unfortunately, we can't live on fat and sugar alone; we need other foods, such as meat, fish and eggs, vegetables, cereals and fruit, to supply all the nutrients that keep us healthy. So, it is not surprising that chocoholics frequently surpass their daily calorie requirements, and therefore put on weight easily. It has been estimated that, next to hard drugs, the three biggest 'crutches' for overstressed humanity are cigarettes, drink and chocolate. What a pity that the least physically harmful of the three is not a low-calorie, full-of-goodness food ... then we could all indulge with a clear conscience and a slim waistline!

Which Choc-Lover Are You?

During our research with chocolate cravers, we found that most sufferers fit into one of six chocoholic 'types', and some span a couple of categories.

Establishing which type of chocoholic you are is the first step towards controlling your chocoholism. That is because each type needs a slightly different version of the basic diet, and also different behavioural and psychological 'exercises' to help break the habits, tensions and thought patterns that are making them fat and miserable.

Below is a guide to the six main categories. At the end of each section you will find a list of questions which you should answer honestly. They will help you decide which diet plan to follow. If your particular problems mean that you fit into two categories, follow the diet plan and 'exercises' which fit in best with your lifestyle and food tastes. (For instance, some women find that they become Premenstrual Cravers just before a period, but need the Comfort Eater diet and lifestyle strategy at other times of the month.)

Before you tackle the questions at the end of each section, read the general information on each type very carefully. As you read, you will start to recognise things about yourself that you may not have acknowledged before. Please, don't feel despondent or 'put down' by this. Remember that acknowledging your fat-making habits and problems is the first step towards doing something about them.

.

Type One: Secret Bingers

Characteristics   The secret binger thinks, sometimes mistakenly, that no one knows about his or her choccy cravings. They sneak into sweet shops out of town to buy their secret supplies of chocs, in the hope that they won't bump into a neighbour or friend. They then hide the stores of chocolate in an unlikely place — a child's toy cupboard, garden shed or airing cupboard — and go back later on to stuff themselves. These binges usually happen when they are tired, emotionally upset, feeling lonely or desperately hungry (e.g. after a day or two trying to follow a crazy diet).

The last thing a secret binger wants to do is admit they have a problem. So, they usually refuse chocolate in a social situation, generally protesting that they are 'on a diet' or 'can't stand the stuff'. They may even refuse chocolate-flavoured puddings or an after-dinner mint on the grounds that chocolate 'doesn't agree' with them, and then go back home and reach for the supply in their secret hiding place.

A secret binger is adept at finding odd places for binges — such as in the loo or parked in a car in a lonely layby. The sad thing is that the binge is not an enjoyable experience — it produces feelings of guilt and often nausea. If they are unable to conquer their furtive chocolate-eating habits, secret bingers can develop very serious problems such as bulimia, and frequently need expert one-to-one or group counselling.

Background   The secret binger is often someone who has been brought up with high expectations of achievement. Weaknesses like over-indulgence in chocolates were probably not tolerated lightly in his or her family. As a child, they may have been expected to do exceptionally well academically or at a sport. They may even have achieved high standards, but never perhaps reached the very top — or maybe they feel that they have passed their 'peak'. Sometimes, the secret binger is someone who is weighed down by family responsibilities and problems — single parents and those with money worries can fall into this category. Many women become secret chocolate bingers when they are faced with domestic problems like bringing up difficult teenage children who don't get on with their father or step-father. Youngsters who are under pressure to do well in exams and men who have been made redundant from work are also at risk.

Questions

1. Is there a secret hoard of chocolate hidden somewhere in your office, home or car?

2. Do you intend to eat it alone?

3. Are you satisfied with what you have achieved in your career and personal relationships?

4. Do you think your parents are (or would be) proud of you?

5. Do you feel that you have to do more than your fair share to keep your family happy?

6. Do you ever feel resentful about the lack of fun, leisure time or sexual satisfaction in your lifestyle?

7. Have you ever followed a low-calorie diet for a few days, then 'pigged-out' on chocolate?

8. Have you ever refused to eat chocolate when out with friends, then had a private orgy afterwards?

9. Do you feel very guilty indeed about your chocoholic habits?

10. Are you keeping this book well hidden so no one realises that you have got a problem?

If you answered 'yes' to most of the questions except numbers 3 and 4, you are a Secret Binger. Your diet and strategy are on page 87.

Type Two: Romantics

Characteristics   Since chocolate has such a powerful effect on the psyche and senses, it is no wonder that it is often used as a love-substitute. The Romantic is a person who is simply not getting the physical and emotional affection and understanding that he or she deserves. So, instead of having a romantic time in bed, a cuddle with a loved one or just a loving conversation, they eat chocolate.

Romantics are often single, unattached and lonely. Or, they can be trapped in a loveless or boring relationship. They often buy expensive and unusual chocolate as a substitute for an expensive and unusual lover. Romantics wake up in the night, usually alone, and fancy an orgy of Mars bars or a quick 'fix' of Kit Kat. Female romantics often go for phallic-shaped choc bars like Toblerone or Cadbury's Flake. Men might choose softer, rounder treats like Cadbury's Creme Eggs or the soft-centred chocs in Quality Street packs.

Background   Romantics tend to undervalue themselves as lovers. Maybe they have had a bad experience, or experiences ... or maybe they have never had a lover. If they have been in a stable relationship, it's usually the Romantic who has put all the hard work into it. They feel that chocolate can take over when romance fails. It is more reliable, easily available, reasonably cheap, and you don't need to use a condom to enjoy it! It doesn't matter how successful the Romantic is in his or her career, they feel a failure in love, and somehow unworthy of being loved. Eating chocolate makes them feel sexy and wanted even if it's only for a very short time.

Questions

1. Do you think you are attractive to the opposite sex? *No*

2. Currently, do you have a caring partner? *No*

3. Do you feel that you get enough cuddles?

4. Do you enjoy choccy treats in the middle of the night? *No*

5. Have you ever consoled yourself with a chocolate-eating orgy after a broken romance? *No*

6. Does the smell of chocolate make you feel sexy? *yes*

7. Are you particularly fond of expensive Swiss or Belgian chocolate? *nope*

8. When you've eaten chocolate, do you feel a sense of satisfaction that is so powerful it is almost sexual? *yes*

9. Do you crave less chocolate when your love-life is going smoothly? (Think about it!) *yes*

10. Do you make jokes about your choc-loving habits? *yes*

If you answered 'no' to questions 1, 2 and 3, but 'yes' to most of the others, then you are a Romantic. Your diet and strategy are on page 109.

Type Three: Comfort Eaters

Characteristics   This is by far the most common type of chocoholic. The Comfort Eater eats chocolate when stressed, lonely, tired or faced with problems. In acute cases, the sufferer will tuck into chocs all day long, rather than deal with the underlying cause or causes of the cravings. For example, a Comfort Eater may be in a high-pressure job with deadlines to meet. When things get tough, they instinctively turn to the chocolate-vending machine, canteen or trolley. Often, Comfort Eaters live alone — students, divorced and separated people for instance. They tend to buy chocolate on a daily basis, rather than hoarding it. You will see highly stressed Comfort Eaters desperately throwing a few choc bars in their trolley at the supermarket check-out point and probably tucking in to one or two in the car park.

Background   Comfort Eaters have usually been given chocolate as a comfort food in childhood, and the habit of eating something sweet and creamy when stressed has stuck. They usually have a pile of problems (possibly no more than other people, but they just seem more), which they find difficult to cope with. There may be no one sympathetic enough to talk to (perhaps partners are unwilling or too busy to help). Because they lack organisation, Comfort Eaters will kid themselves that it is quicker and easier to snack on chocolate than to have a proper meal.

Questions

1. Did your parents give you chocolate as a 'comfort' food when you were a child?

2. Do you think you are overworked, overstressed, overwrought — or even all three?

3. Do your problems seem to get more complicated every day?

4. Are you ever lonely (even if you are living with someone)?

5. Have you ever eaten a chocolate bar while sobbing your heart out?

6. Do you enjoy eating chocs while you watch weepy movies on TV?

7. If someone gives you chocs, do you mean to eat them gradually but wolf the lot down when you feel the blues coming on?

8. Do you eat chocolate while you are waiting (impatiently!) at bus-stops, stations or queuing at the bank?

9. If the washing machine flooded what would you do first — eat a chocolate biscuit or call the plumber?

10. If your partner throws a wobbly, would you rather

go up to your bedroom with a box of chocs than sit down and discuss the situation?

If you answered 'yes' to seven or more of the questions, then you are a Comfort Eater. Your diet plan and strategy are on page 95.

Type Four: Weekend Indulgers

Characteristics   This is the chocoholic who uses every weekend, holiday and outing as an excuse for a sweet treat — or several! Friday night is for stocking up with chocs, from the garage, the supermarket or from the local confectioner's shop on the way home from work. Men tend to favour the garage as a purchasing point for its convenience and macho image. It is fine for a man to buy chocs when he is paying for petrol, too 'feminine' to be seen doing so in a confectionery store or supermarket. The Weekend Indulger will sometimes pretend that this mound of goodies is for 'the kids', but in fact most of it is destined for 'grown-ups'. The Weekend Indulger is also an Easter and Christmas chocolate junkie, even going to the trouble of losing a few pounds before each of these annual eating orgies so they can indulge with a relatively clear conscience. The Weekend Indulger loves chocolate puddings on Sundays (and by way of an excuse explains that this is 'the only day of the week I allow myself to eat them'), chocs for occasions like theatre and cinema outings, and they often give boxes of expensive chocs to other people so they can nibble them too!

Background   Again, childhood behaviour patterns are very important, for the Weekend Indulger usually comes from a family where chocs were considered an important part of family celebrations. The Weekend Indulger continues this family tradition with a vengeance, especially when he or she is having a stressful time, or when they may be in an unsatisfactory relationship. They have to learn that they can have fun without necessarily eating chocs too. They also need plenty of oral gratification, so kisses, cuddles and sensual food are all very important.

Questions

1. Were Easter Eggs and Christmas chocs an important part of your childhood?

2. Do you buy most of your chocs on Fridays or before a holiday or outing?

3. When you go out for a meal, do you feel vaguely disappointed in your evening unless you've enjoyed a choccy dessert from the dessert trolley?

4. After such an evening, are you likely to tuck into a few chocolate biscuits at home before bedtime?

5. Do you ever pretend to buy chocolate for your children, and eat it yourself?

6. Is a trip to the theatre incomplete without a box of chocolates?

7. Do you like to eat chocolate on Sunday afternoon or evening, when you are relaxed and feel that you deserve a treat because it is your day off?

8. Does your partner often bring you chocs as a present?

9. Do you like to eat chocolate slowly, savouring every mouthful?

10. Does the smell and taste of chocolate conjure up happy memories for you?

If you answered 'yes' to seven or more of the questions, you are a Weekend Indulger. Your diet and strategy are on page 115.

Type Five: Sugar Addicts

Characteristics   Sugar Addicts are 'hooked' on sugar, rather like chronic smokers are hooked on nicotine. They obtain most of their daily calories from carbohydrate, using chocolate bars as a 'fix' when they feel tired, hungry or fed up. Dancers, models, actors, students and even sports people can fall into this category. Dancers, particularly, who are terrified of putting on weight, may stop eating conventional meals, grabbing chocolate bars to fill the energy gap. Unfortunately, sugar addiction can be extremely dangerous, leading to long-term health problems.

Background   Pressure is the problem for most Sugar Addicts. They are under pressure to perform, achieve, and keep going, in all circumstances. This pressure may have started back in their childhood or teens, or be self-generated once the Sugar Addict has entered the rat race. The feeling of being on a treadmill is, sadly, increased by their diet. The craving for sugar must be satisfied at all costs (like the craving for a cigarette), but once it has been satisfied, there is only a short respite before another 'fix' is needed. This is because chocolate creates a blood sugar 'high', which is quickly followed by a 'low'. It is a vicious circle of craving which is very hard to break.

Questions

1. Are you in a job which requires very high standards of mental and physical performance?

2. Are you usually too rushed to stop for breakfast and lunch?

3. Do you ever feel weak and wobbly because you have missed several meals?

4. Are you then likely to eat a chocolate bar or sweet snack rather than make time for a proper meal?

5. Are you generally uninterested in gourmet eating?

6. Do you live alone or share a flat with friends?

8. Do you believe that we need a certain amount of sugar each day to keep going?

9. If someone cut off your chocolate supplies completely, would you worry that you could not do your job properly?

10. Do you keep a chocolate bar, or bars, in your handbag, briefcase or work bag for emergencies?

If you answered 'yes' to seven or more of these questions, especially numbers 1, 2, 3 and 4, then you are, or are becoming, a Sugar Addict. Your diet and strategy are on page 122.

Type Six: Premenstrual Cravers

Characteristics   Most chocoholic women have fallen into this category at some time or other. Many become Premenstrual Cravers for a few days every month, when they may find themselves stuffing chocolate bars at very strange times indeed — in the bath, at the hairdressers, waiting outside the school for the children, in the middle of an important meeting at work. At this time, they may even buy brands of chocolate which they do not normally fancy.

Background   Hormonal activity just before a menstrual period can cause tension and even severe depression. One theory is that these symptoms are caused by Vitamin B deficiency. Lack of Vitamin B means that the liver cannot break down the monthly build up of the hormone oestrogen. An excess of oestrogen causes an imbalance of chemicals in the brain and it is thought that too many stimulating chemicals are made and not enough dopamine, which normally has a soothing effect on the body. Adequate levels of B vitamins (particularly Vitamin B6) and magnesium are needed for normal dopamine production. Chocolate contains a relatively high level of magnesium, so that terrible craving for chocs could be your body's way of telling you that your stores are low. Unfortunately, the chocolate is so high in sugar, too, that it will definitely make you feel worse. Better by far to take Vitamin B6 and eat more leafy vegetables and cereals!

Questions

1. Do you feel even more frantic to eat chocolate during the week before your monthly period?

2. Do these cravings strike so fiercely that you have to buy a bar of chocolate immediately, even if it means missing a train or being late for an appointment?

3. Are you more inclined to eat the chocolate quickly than savour it slowly?

4. Are you often accused by your family of being extra touchy at this time of the month?

5. Do you take Vitamin B just before your period?

6. Do you buy special chocs to cheer yourself up?

7. Is the week after your period the only time when you can lose weight?

8. Do you make any extra effort to pamper yourself and relax when you are premenstrual?

9. When trying to slim, have you always had difficulty in curbing your choc-eating habits at this time of the month?

10. Do you also sometimes crave more cigarettes and/or alcohol as well as chocolate?

If you answered 'yes' to most of the questions except numbers 5 and 8, then you are a Premenstrual Craver and you should follow the diet and strategy on page 102.

5

Chocs Away?

Imagine being told to eat ten bars of chocolate every day and keep the wrappers piled up on your office desk for everyone to see. That is the kind of treatment that is recommended for chocoholics by some behaviour therapists. Their argument is that this kind of therapy will, eventually, make the sufferer give up. Personally, I am pretty sure that it would make them throw up ... but giving up is something else!

Even the shame of knowing that other people are disgusted by their behaviour is not enough to help severe chocoholics stop. It simply makes them switch to eating chocolate in secret, which can cause all kinds of physical and psychological problems including obesity and depression.

After talking to many, many chocolate 'junkies', I am convinced that it is much more sensible to cut down on your chocolate intake and learn to enjoy it in small quantities. You can only do this by following a good diet plan which is specifically designed to keep your blood sugar level high and to make you feel in great shape.

A chronic sufferer who expanded from a size 12 to a size 22 after becoming hooked on chocolates told me, 'Chocoholism is the same as being an alcoholic but without Alcoholics Anonymous to help. I even tried the Samaritans, who were kind but didn't know much. There's acupuncture, if you can afford it, and doctors aren't much help. Mine recommended anti-depressants!' She recovered after following a vitamin-and-mineral-rich diet for six months, and now sticks to the same basic plan. She has also managed to lose 3 stone in weight and is still losing.

Well-known chocoholics include superstar Cher, Nina Myscow, Lulu and Elizabeth Taylor.

Cher, world-famous singer and actress, loves m&ms and is very partial to Häagen-Dazs chocolate ice cream. She is, however, very interested in nutrition and has worked out a diet with her nutritional adviser, Dr Robert Haas. This diet keeps her blood sugar level high all day so she does not get choccy cravings too often. She also maintains that exercise is a tremendous help. It could well be that the endorphins, a group of chemicals manufactured in the brain, which are produced by rigorous exercise give a similar 'high' to that experienced after a chocolate 'fix'. Exercise is certainly helpful in alleviating stress and maximising energy levels. Cher still has occasional binges which are usually triggered by stress or exhaustion. Her diet and exercise control her chocoholism but will never beat it. During the making of the movie *The Witches of Eastwick*, she admits to having chocolate orgies with fellow actress Michelle Pfeiffer who is also a choc fan.

Nina Myscow has tried all kinds of chocoholic cures. She says, 'My mother used to stuff food in my mouth to shut me up. I graduated from biscuits to doughnuts to the sensual pleasure of chocolate. By the time I reached my thirties, I was an expert. I have gorged myself on bars of Cadbury's Whole Nut and stuffed myself silly with chocolate-covered doughnuts.

'My worst-ever crisis was when I came home from a holiday in West Africa and bought two huge slabs of chocolate when I changed planes at Geneva Airport. I only meant to eat one on the plane but found myself sitting next to a wizened Japanese businessman instead of a handsome hunk. I ate both through sheer disappointment and felt even worse.

'In my time, I have tried crazy crash diets, hypnosis, you name it. But the only thing that works is to eat sensibly, take exercise and learn to enjoy chocolate when you have it. Now, I can eat one perfectly formed white Belgian chocolate each week and relish every mouthful. I can also go into a newsagent and just buy the papers, a can of diet coke and a small pack of nuts and raisins. I wouldn't say that I am cured, but I definitely have the problem well under control.'

The singer Lulu inherited her chocoholism from her mum, Betty. Lulu agrees that there is no such thing as a cure for the affliction and declares that she wouldn't want one. 'I'd hate to think that I could never again sit down to my favourite, French-style breakfast of a croissant with a piece of rich, dark chocolate,' she says. 'So, I now allow for it in my daily diet. I think you've got to look at the whole you when you're trying to improve your life. Take a step back and try and work out what is making you so dependent on chocolate. I've found that meditation helps me in everything from dealing with work problems, to planning what to eat.'

Here is a round-up of six ways of controlling chocoholism and the pros and cons of each method:

1. *Quitting 'Cold Turkey'* This method is often used successfully by smokers. They make a New Year's resolution to quit on 1 January and do so - just like that! It only works for smokers if they have prepared themselves mentally for the day when they quit. This

includes reading up everything they can lay their hands on about the dangers of smoking, ear-marking the precise items they will buy with the cash they save, and giving themselves other rewards like holidays, outings and luxuries. Problems arise when they hit a stressful situation where they cannot turn to their usual 'prop'. That's why so many former smokers become sweet-oholics instead, put on weight and go right back to smoking again!

Chocolate addiction is just as complex as nicotine addiction, but is related to comfort and guilt as well as stress and physical cravings. Only someone with the most amazing willpower could give up a six-Mars-a-day habit just like that! In fact, if anyone reading this book has been able to do it, I would very much like to hear from them (my address is on page 236).

Trying to give up chocolates completely is quite dangerous because it frequently leads to a very bad binge once the next 'crisis' (whether it's a lovers' tiff or something far more serious) occurs. What does work well is to cut out chocolate completely for a week or a couple of weeks, while altering your eating habits. The discipline of doing so gives you a boost, and you still have the promise of chocolate to come at a later date, even though it will be in smaller quantities. Meanwhile, good nutrition is helping you to arm yourself to eat chocolate in moderation. This method worked very well with volunteers who tried out the various programmes on *The Chocolate Diet*.

2. *Cutting down* If your body is used to a massive amount of sugar each day, you will probably feel faint and ill for a few days if you try to cut down. Again, the only answer is to change your eating habits at the same time. You must make sure that you eat regularly, and have alternative snack foods available. The diet on page 151 (How to Stay Slim) can help if you are not very overweight, but feel that a healthier diet, and fewer chocs, would be good for you. It will, it will!

3. *Hypnotism and acupuncture* These treatments may help addicts cope with symptoms like depression and guilt but they will not turn a confirmed chocoholic into a choc-hater. You must want to cut down before

these can help. One acupuncturist told me, 'I get people with all kinds of cravings asking for treatment, including chocolate cravers. But, acupuncuture is not a cure-all and I can only offer a treatment to supplement nutrition therapy.' A hypnotist who has had terrific success with smokers says, 'Chocoholism is different. I once had a patient who weighed 25 stone and ate three boxes of chocs and ten bars of chocolate every day. She was told by her doctor that she would probably have to be brought into hospital unless she could control her chocolate intake because of complications caused by her weight problems. She had high blood pressure and a heart murmur. The fear of hospitalisation made her want to beat chocoholism, so we worked out a plan which involved a hospital diet and hypnotism. The hypnotism did help, but I'm sure it was her own fear and the diet which really made her cut down. She was very receptive to my therapy, and that is absolutely essential if it is going to work. So far, she has managed to lose 3 stone, and we are still working well together, but it is a slow process.'

4. *Behaviour therapy* Like hypnotism and acupuncture, behaviour therapy can only be part of a chocoholic's cutdown campaign. However, it is a very useful part. While I would not advise the type of therapy described in the first paragraph of this chapter, I do think that monitoring how, when and why you eat your chocs is very helpful. Check through the points listed on pages 206-209 for your own behaviour therapy guide.

5. *Crash dieting* This can help you lose a lot of weight very fast, but you will put it back on again even more rapidly. Once you come off a diet that is below around 1,750 calories for men, or 1,500 for women, your body is programmed to store any extra calories. As a chocoholic, these calories are likely to be in the form of your favourite high-fat, high-sugar treat. So, you'll end up eating more chocolate, not less.

6. *Exercise* The benefits of exercise are well-documented, but for those who have not experienced them it is worth giving a few reminders here. Exercise

can help strengthen your heart, reduce blood pressure and prevent stress. It can also help you maintain your correct body weight and cut your appetite. The feeling of well-being produced by exercise is an effective substitute for 'props' such as nicotine, alcohol and chocolate. All the chocoholics we worked with while researching this book found that regular exercise (a minimum of 20 minutes' aerobic exercise - i.e. swimming, jogging, dancing) helped improve their self-image and made them a whole lot happier. However, exercise alone is unlikely to help overweight chocoholics cure their cravings or lose any weight.

6

The Chocolate Diet: Six Plans that Really Work

*H*ere they are, the six diet plans that can turn chocolate cravers into calm, controlled, slim people.

By completing the quiz in Chapter Four, you should already have discovered which kind of chocoholic you are. If you feel that you fall into two categories, try one plan first, and see how it goes. All the plans have one thing in common: they include regular, filling meals that keep your blood sugar level high, so you are never hungry.

Our researchers found that learning to eat

regularly was the very first step towards conquering their addiction. While you continue to neglect your body by missing meals, snatching empty snacks and following crash diets, you will never cure your chocoholism. Emotional and behavioural triggers that precipitate an attack are hard enough to conquer without the additional burden of acute, tummy-rumbling hunger pangs.

So, please follow your diet faithfully, without missing any meals at all. If you hate eating breakfast, you can pack it up and take it with you to work. Don't be tempted to miss out on that first, vital meal of the day.

THE FIRST WEEK

Please stop eating chocolate altogether for the very first week of your diet. This is important because it is a vital part of learning to control your cravings. On subsequent weeks, you will be given an allowance of chocolate, chosen from the list on page 213 or the recipes in Chapter 9.

Clear out any hoards of chocolate which you may have stashed away in the house. Give them to a neighbour, your mother-in-law or throw them away. Make sure there are no hidden chocs in the freezer, in the glove compartment of your car or under the bed. If other members of the family are chocolate eaters, ask them to keep the chocs out of your sight just for the first week of your diet.

FREE VEGETABLE LIST

All six diets allow unlimited amounts of certain, very low-calorie vegetables. Pile them up on your plate but do not add butter or margarine or salad dressings other than lemon juice, vinegar and herbs. It is important that you munch your way through as much as you can of these 'free' veggies — they supply valuable vitamins and minerals which will help you in your fight against chocolate addiction. Here is the list:

asparagus	fennel
beansprouts	gherkins
broccoli	leeks
Brussels sprouts	lettuce
cabbage	mushrooms
cauliflower	mustard and cress
celery	peppers (red and green)
chicory	radishes
Chinese leaves	runner beans
chives	shallots
courgettes	spinach
cucumber	spring onions (scallions)
curly kale	tomatoes (canned or fresh)
endive	watercress

MEN Please add around 300 calories to your diet plan by having 2 extra slices of wholemeal bread with a little low-fat spread or a couple of small rolls plus 1/2 pint extra beer or lager. If you are tee-total, have a small potato instead. If you are in a 'heavy' job, such as construction work, please add an extra 100g meat or fish, or 50g low-fat cheese as well.

Diet for Secret Bingers

DAILY ALLOWANCES $^1/_2$ pint (275ml) semi-skimmed milk, water and mineral water. Drink lots of water — about 6–8 glasses daily. Try to avoid tea and coffee — no more than 2 weak cups of tea daily. Try herbal tea instead. Take a multivitamin capsule every day.

FREE VEGETABLES Eat as much as you like from the 'free' vegetable list. You can boil or steam veggies, or serve them as salads. Do not add butter or margarine, and use lemon juice, vinegar and herb dressings on salads.

CHOCOLATE None the first week, sorry. This is the start of the rest of your life. Once you have your blood sugar level under control, and are psychologically adjusted to living without your chocolate 'crutch', you can gradually reintroduce the chocs. Your allowance for Week Two and subsequent weeks is 150 calories daily (check the chart towards the end of the book for the calorie count of your favourite chocs).

- Try to halve the amount of cigarettes you normally smoke
- Cut down on alcohol to the amount allowed under Treats
- Do not add salt when cooking. Use herbs, lemon juice and garlic instead.

STRATEGY

1. The act of clearing out your choccy hoards is especially important for you. Starting with a 'clean slate' will help you stick to the diet. You could be surprised at how much this one act of control will help you. Reward yourself afterwards with a good long soak in a scented bath. You can tell someone about it if you like, but don't be surprised or put off if they are less than hopeful about your chances of sticking to the diet

— it may be in their interest to keep you fat! Remember, this is for you.

2. Confession time: write down a list of things you are worried about, fear or are unhappy with in your life. Secret chocoholism is often a sneaky way of avoiding looking at other problems in your life. If you have a good friend (not a relative) who you can discuss this with, do so. Talking it through will help you cope. If you prefer, keep the list private — just writing it is a way of facing things, instead of burying them. Don't forget that you can write to me, at the address on page 236, if you wish. Where problems are very serious, please do seek the help of a trained counsellor. You can get a list at your public library or Citizen's Advice Bureau, or we can help.

3. Treat time: sneaking off for a chocolate binge is now a thing of the past for you ... we hope! Instead, try sneaking off for one of these treats: a facial, massage or manicure; a swim in the local pool; a window-shopping expedition; a walk in the park with a good book for

company, and fruit to eat; a browse round a music store.

4. Walk briskly for at least 20 minutes each day. This will help speed up your metabolism, and make you feel less hungry.

5. Go swimming or try some other relaxing exercise once a week — dancing, skating and yoga are also excellent. The exercises in Chapter 7 have been specially devised for chocoholics — try them.

WEEK ONE

EVERY DAY Eat *one* Breakfast, *two* Light Meals, and *one* Main Meal, plus *one* Treat. You can eat them when you like, but please do not leave long gaps between eating. Have a large glass of water before each meal and plenty of water between meals.

BREAKFASTS (250 calories)
• 50g any unsweetened cereal, milk from allowance, 1 chopped banana, small glass fruit juice

- Sandwich of 2 slices wholemeal bread with 2 tbsp cottage cheese, sliced tomato, a few grapes, 1 satsuma
- 1 slice wholemeal toast topped with grilled tomatoes, 1 size 3 poached egg, small glass fruit juice
- 1 large slice of melon sprinkled with 2 tbsp cottage cheese, 12g mixed nuts, small glass unsweetened orange juice, 1 diet yoghurt

LIGHT MEALS (350 calories each)

Jacket Potatoes Make a huge salad from the 'free' list (page 86), add 200g jacket potato and one of these toppings, and an apple or an orange:

- 2 tbsp baked beans
- $1/2$ carton natural yoghurt
- 100g carton low-calorie coleslaw

Salads Make a huge mixed salad with vegetables from 'free' list (page 86) and serve it with one of these choices, and a medium banana:

- 200g chicken leg, no skin, grilled or roast, 1 apple or orange
- 100g grilled or steamed fish, no sauces, 2 small

boiled potatoes, 1 small banana
• 1 small carton cottage cheese, 2 tbsp sweetcorn, 2 chopped apricots, 1 slice wholemeal bread

Sandwiches 2 slices wholemeal bread with salad from 'free' list and one of these fillings, and an apple or pear:
• 50g tuna-in-brine with lemon juice
• 2 tbsp cottage cheese
• 50g peeled prawns
• 25g lean ham or chicken

Soups
• 1 tin slimmer's soup, any flavour, 1 slice wholemeal bread, 1 carton low-fat fruit yoghurt, 1 apple
• Home-made vegetable soup (use vegetables from 'free' list) with wholemeal croutons, 1 slice toast topped with tomatoes, 12g grated Edam cheese, 1 pear

MAIN MEALS (400 calories each) Don't forget to add piles of 'free' vegetables and salad.
• 1 large slice of melon, 75g canned sardines on 2 slices wholemeal toast, grilled tomatoes, watercress, 1 orange

- 100g grilled liver, thin gravy with 2 tbsp fresh orange juice added, 2 boiled potatoes, 2 tbsp sweetcorn, 1 banana
- 125g lamb chop, thin gravy, 75g mashed potato made with milk from allowance, 1 pear or 2 apricots, slice of bread
- Any supermarket ready-meal of 350 calories or less and a small roll, with 1 piece fresh fruit afterwards
- 125g grilled herring or tinned pilchards, 2 small boiled potatoes, 1 serving low-fat mousse
- 1 well-grilled beefburger, 2 tbsp sweetcorn, 200g jacket potato, 100g strawberries or raspberries
- 75g any lean meat, thin gravy, 2 small chunks roast potato, 1 small wholemeal roll
- 75g (cooked weight) wholemeal pasta or wholegrain rice with one of the following toppings and an apple and orange to follow:
- 100g prawns with tomatoes, garlic, herbs
- 50g chopped ham with tin of slimmer's mushroom soup
- 100g chicken breast with tin of slimmer's chicken soup

TREATS (100 calories) Choose *one* each day.

• 1 glass dry wine

• 2 pub-measure 'short' drinks with low-calorie mixers (use soda or tonic — not sweet-tasting soft drinks)

• $1/2$ pint beer or lager

• 2 crispbreads topped with 2 tbsp cottage cheese, sliced gherkins or 1 tsp sweet pickle

• 1 mug Batchelors Slim a Soup with small slice wholemeal bread

WEEK TWO and subsequent weeks

You may now have 150 calories of chocolate from the Calorie Guide to Your Favourite Chocs on page 213. You may also have one 200-calorie dessert or drink from the recipes listed in Chapter 9 (pages 173-204) each day.

Diet for Comfort Eaters

DAILY ALLOWANCES $^1/_2$ pint (275ml) semi-skimmed milk for your tea and coffee, unlimited water, mineral water. Please cut down on those cups of tea, substituting herb teas, and more water.

FREE VEGETABLES You can have as much as you like of the vegetables on the 'free' list (page 86). Serve them lightly boiled or steamed, or as salad. Do not add butter or other fat. Make your own salad dressing using lemon juice, vinegar, black pepper, herbs and garlic. Avoid salt; do not use it in cooking or sprinkle it on your food.

CHOCOLATE 200 calories daily in the second week, decreasing to 150 calories daily in the third week. Buy your chocolate allowance every day, do not hoard it. When you buy it, put it into a tin immediately. Eat your chocolate allowance when things are going well, not when they are going badly. Do not eat chocs when you have had a row with your kids or spouse, nibble them when you are having a jolly time. Choose your chocs from the calorie guide on page 213 or from the recipes in Chapter 9.

STRATEGY

1. Stress is one of the things that is making you eat more chocolate than you should. You can get the same 'high' from exercise as you do from chocs. While you are following the diet, please attend a health club, gym or aerobics class at least three times weekly. You need the kind of exercise that will make you feel out of breath for around 20 minutes, three times a week. An exercise bike at home can help too. But cheaper and just as effective is to run up and down stairs, or use the bottom stair for some 'stepping' exercises.

2. Every day, make a list of all the things you have to do both for work, yourself and your family. As they are accomplished, tick them off. Don't let worries pile on top of you. Try to deal with problems logically. Consult

your partner or a friend if you are worried about something. If this is impossible, talk to your doctor or a counsellor. Write to me at the address on page 236, if you need any advice that is not contained in this book.

3. If you live alone or feel lonely even though you live with someone else, it is always a good idea to make contact with organisations in your local community. Doing some charity work, or joining a club, or going to an evening class will give you a new angle on life. For, even if you are a busy career person (and many chocoholic comfort eaters are high-flyers who boss others around all day), a change is as good as a rest.

4. Talk to someone new every day. That doesn't mean chatting up someone at random, but it means having a pleasant word with someone who's non-threatening like a shop assistant, taxi driver or work colleague who you haven't spoken to before.

5. Try swimming, skating, dancing or a yoga class each week, and do the special exercises in Chapter 7.

6. When you feel an urge to eat chocs, have a long glass of water, phone a friend, and if you still feel that you must eat a choc, have one of the emergency snacks or treats listed below instead.

WEEK ONE

EVERY DAY Choose *one* Breakfast, *one* Light Meal, *one* Main Meal, *and* two Treats.

BREAKFASTS (250 calories)
- 1 slice wholemeal toast topped with mashed banana and 1 tsp honey, small glass fruit juice
- 25g any unsweetened cereal, milk from allowance, 1 apple, two crispbreads with a little low-fat spread
- 1 egg, boiled or poached, 1 slice wholemeal toast, small glass fruit juice
- 100g tinned apricots or figs topped with 1 tbsp muesli and 1 tbsp natural yoghurt
- 2 tbsp sweetcorn, 75g mushrooms poached in chicken stock, grilled tomatoes, 1 grilled vegeburger, 2 crispbreads

LIGHT MEALS (350 calories)

Cooked Meals Any supermarket ready-meal of 350 calories (check pack) or under, with a huge pile of vegetables and/or salad from the 'free' list.

Jacket Potatoes Make a huge salad from 'free' list (page 86), add a 200g jacket potato and one of these toppings:
• 4 tbsp baked beans
• 1 carton natural yoghurt
• 100g carton cottage cheese

Salads Make a huge salad using vegetables from 'free' list (page 86), and add one of these:
• 200g chicken leg, no skin, grilled or roast, 1 apple or orange, crusty roll
• 150g grilled or steamed fish, 2 boiled potatoes, 1 small banana
• 1 small carton cottage cheese, 2 tbsp sweetcorn, 2 chopped apricots, 1 slice wholemeal bread, 1 banana

Sandwiches 2 slices of wholemeal bread with salad from

'free' list (page 86) and one of these fillings:
• 100g tuna in brine with lemon juice
• 50g lean ham or chicken

Soup Use Weight Watchers soups from Heinz as a base and add extra vegetables from 'free' list (page 86), plus 50g chopped chicken, ham or tuna, 1 small wholemeal roll

MAIN MEALS (400 calories) Don't forget to add piles of 'free' vegetables (page 86) and salads.
• 75g (cooked weight) wholemeal pasta or wholegrain rice with one of the following toppings and an apple and orange to follow:
• 100g prawns with tomatoes, garlic, herbs
• 50g chopped ham with tin of slimmer's mushroom soup
• 100g chicken breast with tin of slimmer's chicken soup
• 1 well-grilled beefburger, 2 tbsp sweetcorn, grilled tomatoes, 1 slice wholemeal bread, 1 large banana chopped and served topped with a little milk from allowance and 12g mixed nuts

- Any ready meal of 350 calories or less
- 75g any lean roast meat, thin gravy, 75g peas, 75g carrots, 75g chunks roast potato, 1 apple or orange
- 200g grilled chicken leg, no skin, 200g jacket potato, 1 small banana
- Casserole of 150g chicken or fish cooked in 1 tin low-calorie slimmer's soup, with sliced onions and peppers, 75g potato, mashed with milk from allowance, 1 carton low-calorie fromage frais
- Takeaway meal of $1/2$ portion medium thin pizza or 1 KFC dinner

TREATS OR EMERGENCY SNACKS (50 calories each)
Choose *one* each day.
- $1/2$ glass dry wine, topped up with soda, and a few grapes
- 2 crispbreads topped with 1 tbsp cottage cheese and chopped gherkin
- 1 small banana
- 10 grapes
- 1 slice low-calorie bread topped with salad from 'free' list

WEEK TWO and subsequent weeks

Add 200 calories of chocolate each day decreasing to 150 calories in Week Three and until you reach your goal weight. You may also add one 200-calorie dessert or drink from the recipe section each day. But, please make sure you eat it when things are going well!

Diet for Premenstrual Cravers

This diet should be followed for one or two weeks before or during a menstrual period.

DAILY ALLOWANCES 1/2 pint (275ml) semi-skimmed milk for your tea and coffee, unlimited water and mineral water. Try to replace as many cups of tea and coffee as you can with water or herbal teas.

FREE VEGETABLES Eat as much as you like from the 'free' vegetable list (page 86). Do not add butter or low-fat spread, and use just lemon juice, garlic, herbs and vinegar to make a salad dressing.

CHOCOLATE On the second week of your diet, you can have up to 100 calories of chocolate each day from the list on page 213. If you like, save it up for a larger amount, say twice a week. However, if you follow the diet correctly and are not a serious chocoholic you may find that you no longer experience choccy cravings at all.

- During the week before your period, and the week of your period, take two Vitamin B6 capsules and four Evening Primrose Oil capsules each day.
- Do not add salt when cooking. Instead, use herbs, lemon juice and garlic if you like it.

STRATEGY

1. Walk briskly for at least 20 minutes each day. This will help ease tension as well as speed up your metabolism.

2. Do deep breathing exercises in front of your mirror every morning. Start by exhaling slowly through your mouth, then inhale through your nose. Repeat

ten times, before facing the problems of the day.

3. Beat tension headaches with exercises for your shoulders and neck: try backwards arm-swings, hunching then relaxing your shoulders, putting your right hand over your right shoulder and trying to touch it with your left hand, then repeating to the left.

4. Try acupressure: place your middle fingers in the hollow at the side of your head just by your brow bone. Press firmly, hold for a count of six, then relax. This really does help soothe away headaches, so try it before you take a pain-killer; you may not need one.

   Have a go at this one too: kneel on a cushion, join your hands together with your fingers back to back, fingertips pointing towards your tummy. Let your relaxed fingers press into the centre of your tummy, below the ribs, above the navel. Now lean gently forward and exhale. Raise yourself upright as you inhale. Repeat six times, then have a good stretch as you get up. This is a good exercise to help relieve feelings of depression or anxiety.

5. Go swimming once or twice a week or join a yoga or dance class. Swimming is wonderfully relaxing and also exercises every part of your body, but gently. So, it is the perfect sport. Yoga and dance also help beat tension. Don't push yourself into an aerobics class, or go jogging — both can be too exhausting for comfort!

6. When you feel low, give yourself a treat — a scented bath, a walk in the park, a low-calorie lunch with a friend. Don't mope ... you can cope!

Now choose five 250-calorie meals each day from the lists below, plus *one* treat (including alcohol!). If you like, you can lump a couple of the meals together, but it is best to spread your food allowance out ... especially in those dangerous days just before your period.

CEREAL MEALS

- $1/2$ grapefruit, 50g any unsweetened cereal topped with a medium banana, milk from allowance
- 1 Weetabix, milk from allowance, 2 crispbreads topped with a little low-fat spread, 1 carton low-fat fruit yoghurt
- 25g porridge made up with water and milk from allowance, 1 apple, 1 crispbread topped with 1 Kraft Cheese triangle, small glass fruit juice
- 100g figs canned in syrup, sprinkled with 2 tbsps unsweetened muesli and topped with 1 carton natural yoghurt

FISH MEALS Use 'free' vegetables (page 86) or salad, plus one of the following:
- 150g any grilled or steamed fish, 2 boiled potatoes
- 125g grilled herring, 2 crispbreads with low-fat spread
- Any fishy ready-meal of 250 calories, a few grapes or 2 apricots
- 100g any shellfish, 1 slice wholemeal bread, 1 apple

JACKET POTATO MEALS Bake a 200g jacket potato, and serve with a huge portion of salad or vegetables from the 'free' list (page 86), plus one of these toppings:

- 3 tbsp cottage cheese or baked beans
- 12g grated Edam cheese mixed with tinned tomatoes
- 1 carton natural yoghurt with chives

MEAT MEALS Use unlimited 'free' vegetables (page 86), boiled or steamed, with one of the following choices:

- 150g lean chump chop, with thin gravy
- 200g chicken joint, grilled or roast, no skin, thin gravy
- 75g any lean roast meat, thin gravy, 1 boiled potato
- 1 well-grilled beefburger, 1 small (125g) tin baked beans, 1 apple

SALAD MEALS Make yourself a huge salad using vegetables from 'free' list (page 86). As well as lettuce and tomatoes, try raw cauliflower, spinach, cold cooked green beans and courgettes, etc. Now add one of these choices:

- 100g chicken (no skin)
- 2 tbsp sweetcorn, 1 apple, 1 small carton cottage cheese
- 100g any white fish, grilled or steamed, 2 small boiled potatoes
- 200g jacket potato, 12g grated Edam cheese
- 75g lean ham, 1 small wholemeal roll

SANDWICH MEALS 2 thin slices wholemeal bread with salad from 'free' list (page 86) and one of these:

- 25g grated Edam cheese, 1 apple
- 3 tbsp cottage cheese, 1 orange
- 100g tuna-in-brine, 1 pear
- 50g chicken (no skin), 2 plums
- 3 tbsp baked beans, 1 rasher chopped grilled lean bacon
- 1 large banana, chopped with lemon juice

TREATS (100 calories) Choose *one* each day.

- 1 glass dry wine
- 2 pub-measure 'short' drinks with low-calorie mixers

- $1/2$ pint beer or lager
- 12g unsalted mixed nuts
- 1 large slice wholemeal bread with a little low-fat spread
- 1 large banana
- 1 carton low-calorie fromage frais or yoghurt with 1 medium digestive biscuit

Diet for Romantics

DAILY ALLOWANCES Water and mineral water. $1/2$ pint (275ml) skimmed milk for your tea and coffee.

FREE VEGETABLES Eat as much as you like from the 'free' vegetable list given (page 86). Do not add butter or low-fat spread, and use just lemon juice, garlic, herbs and vinegar mixed together for a salad dressing.

CHOCOLATE After the first, non-choc week, you are in for a treat. For, three times weekly, you may 'spend' 300 calories on chocolate. This is a *lot*. Select your chocs from the list on page 213 or the recipes in Chapter 9. Make sure that you shop no more, and no less, than three times a week. Enjoy the occasion and do not feel guilty about it.

STRATEGY

1. Make a list of all the good things about you — physical, intellectual, everything. Keep it somewhere handy and carry on reading it!

2. Make another list of things that normally 'trigger' a chocolate-craving attack. Study it carefully and see if there is any way in which you can avoid these things, or face them differently.

3. During the diet you must have a personal treat every single day. This can be anything that gives you pleasure — from an hour with a favourite magazine, to a long, scented bath or an evening in with a weepy video. And, yes, you may eat chocolate while you indulge — as long as it is from your allowance (see above).

4. If you feel an uncontrollable urge to splurge on chocs coming on, deal with it by (a) drinking two or three glasses of water, (b) making a phone call to someone you love or makes you laugh, (c) going for a brisk walk, or doing a work-out.

5. During your diet, it is advisable to practise the exercises in Chapter 7, or to go swimming several times a week. You are the kind of person who enjoys sensual pleasures so have the occasional massage or sauna, and go to bed with a good, erotic book plus chocs from your allowance.

WEEK ONE
EVERY DAY Eat one Breakfast, one Light Meal, one Main Meal and one Treat.

BREAKFASTS (250 calories)
• 1 slice wholemeal toast, 1 size 3 poached egg, grilled tomato, watercress
• 1 large banana chopped up on top of 50g unsweetened cereal, with milk from allowance

- 1 rasher well-grilled streaky bacon, 50g sweetcorn, 2 crispbreads with a little low-fat spread, 1 small glass unsweetened apple or orange juice
- fruit salad of $1/2$ medium melon, 1 small chopped banana, 2 fresh apricots, 2 tbsp yoghurt, 1 tbsp mixed nuts

LUNCHES (350 calories)

Meals on Toast Top 2 slices wholemeal toast with one of the following:

- Lots of grilled tomatoes sprinkled with 50g grated Edam cheese
- 1 small (125g) can baked beans, tomatoes, watercress, 1 apple
- $1/2$ large can Weight Watchers from Heinz Spaghetti, 1 small banana
- 100g mushrooms poached in chicken stock, 1 carton low-fat fruit yoghurt, and 1 apple to follow

Salads Eat unlimited salad vegetables from your 'free' list (page 86) and choose one of the following accompaniments:

- 200g chicken leg, no skin, 200g jacket potato
- 75g drained sardines, lemon juice, 1 low-fat fruit yoghurt, 1 small roll
- 75g lean ham or smoked salmon, 1 slice wholemeal bread with low-fat spread, 1 large banana

Sandwiches 2 large slices wholemeal bread, salad from 'free' list (page 86) and one of these fillings:
- 100g tuna-in-brine
- 1 sliced hard-boiled egg, 1 tbsp low-cal mayonnaise
- 100g cottage cheese with chopped gherkins and an apple to follow

SUPPERS (400 calories)
- 1 large slice melon, 250g grilled trout or herring, huge salad from 'free' list, 1 small wholemeal roll, 1 pear
- $1/2$ grapefruit with artificial sweetener, 75g lean lamb chop, thin gravy, huge pile of vegetables from 'free' list, 1 potato, 1 scoop vanilla ice cream with 100g strawberries or raspberries
- Any supermarket ready-meal under 450 calories with huge pile of 'free' vegetables and salad

- Slimmer's soup, any flavour, any Bird's Eye Fish in Sauce meal, with vegetables and salad from 'free' list, 1 small banana, apple or pear
- Mixed grill of well-grilled beefburger, 100g mushrooms cooked in chicken stock, grilled tomatoes, watercress, 1 grilled low-fat sausage, 3 tbsp baked beans. Add a huge mixed salad from 'free' list, 1 apple
- *Starter* of sliced tomatoes, 1oz (25g) cubed Edam cheese, chopped chives, with dressing of chopped garlic, vinegar and herbs; *main course* of 100g chicken breast cooked in tin of low-calorie chicken soup, with vegetables from 'free' list; *dessert* of baked apple with 2 squirts of aerosol cream. Yum!
- 75g any roast meat, thin gravy, 75g chunks roast potato, huge helping of 'free' vegetables, red fruit salad (1 sliced red apple, a few redcurrants, raspberries and strawberries) with 2 tbsp natural yoghurt

TREATS (100 calories) Choose *one* each day.
- 1 glass dry wine
- 2 pub-measure 'short' drinks with low-calorie mixers

- $1/2$ pint beer or lager
- 1 large banana
- 1 digestive biscuit

WEEK TWO and subsequent weeks
Add your 300-calorie chocolate allowance just *three* times each week. Enjoy it without feeling guilty. Make sure you nibble each mouthful slowly. Alternatively include the recipes on page 173 onwards in your chocolate allowance, making sure you do not exceed your daily 300-calorie total.

Diet for Weekend Indulgers

This diet allows 1,350 calories on weekdays and 1,600 calories on Saturdays and Sundays.

DAILY ALLOWANCES $1/2$ pint (275ml) semi-skimmed milk for your tea and coffee, unlimited water and mineral water.

FREE VEGETABLES You can eat as much as you like from the 'free' vegetable list (page 86). You can boil or steam vegetables, or eat them raw. Do not use butter or margarine, and make your own dressing using lemon juice, vinegar, herbs and garlic.

• There is an alcohol allowance for weekends only.
• Do not add salt to cooking or sprinkle it on food.

STRATEGY

1. Make a list of the places where you normally buy chocolate — the supermarket, garage or paper shop. Now, relax and imagine yourself going into each of these places without buying chocolate. Do this exercise every single day.

2. Always carry fresh fruit in your car or bag, and eat it before going into a shop or during moments of tension.

3. When you have chocs in the house, make sure they

are kept out of sight in a tin on top of a cupboard.

4. One of your problems is that you associate pleasure and treats with eating chocolates. So, every day give yourself a treat that doesn't involve eating, such as listening to music, reading a book, having a manicure or hair-do.

5. When you go to a film or concert, make sure you eat a good meal before the show. Don't take chocs with you. Sit tight in the interval!

6. You are a sensual person, so indulge in an occasional massage, using scented oils. It is fun to try this with a partner, especially if going to a salon seems too expensive.

7. Get out into the fresh air at weekends. Take up a sport like golf, tennis, or just walk. Contrary to what most people think, exercise helps stop that choccy craving. Aim for 20 minutes of aerobic (swimming, cycling, exercise class) exercise every week.

WEEKDAYS

Choose *one* Breakfast, *one* Light Meal, *one* Main Meal and *one* Treat. Between meals, nibble anything you like from the 'free' vegetable list (page 86).

BREAKFASTS (250 calories)

- 25g any unsweetened cereal, milk from allowance, 1 large banana
- 1 size 3 egg, boiled or poached, 1 slice wholemeal toast with a little low-fat spread, small glass fruit juice
- 1 slice melon, 1 slice wholemeal toast topped with 75g mushrooms, poached in chicken stock sprinkled with 12g grated Edam cheese, 1 apple
- 2 Weetabix, milk from allowance, a few grapes and raisins, small glass orange juice

LIGHT MEALS (350 calories)

Salads Make a huge salad with vegetables from the 'free' list (page 86) and serve with one of these choices:

- 200g chicken leg, no skin, grilled or roast, 1 apple or orange, crusty roll

- 150g steamed or grilled fish, 1 small boiled potato, 1 banana
- 1 small carton cottage cheese, 2 tbsp sweetcorn, 2 chopped apricots, 1 slice wholemeal bread, 1 banana

Sandwiches 2 slices wholemeal bread with salad from 'free' list (page 86) and one of these fillings:
- 1 chopped banana with lemon juice
- 3 tsp peanut butter
- 2 cold, chopped chipolata sausages
- 1 chopped apple with 12g mixed nuts and 1 dsp low-fat mayonnaise

Soups
- 1 tin slimmer's soup, any flavour, 1 slice wholemeal bread, 1 carton low-fat fruit yoghurt
- Home-made vegetable soup (use vegetables from 'free' list) with wholemeal croutons, 1 slice toast topped with tomatoes, 1 apple, 1 orange

MAIN MEALS (450 calories)
Don't forget to pile on the 'free' salads and vegetables.

- Any supermarket ready-meal of 400 calories or less with 1 apple, orange or small banana to follow
- 75g (cooked weight) wholemeal pasta or wholegrain rice with one of the following toppings plus 1 small wholemeal roll and an apple or orange to follow:
  - 75g prawns with tomatoes, herbs, garlic
  - 50g chopped ham with tin of slimmer's mushroom soup
- 100g liver, grilled with thin gravy, 1 rasher streaky bacon, grilled, 1 beef chipolata sausage, grilled, 75g mashed potato, 100g mushrooms poached in water, 1 potato, grilled tomatoes
- 200g chicken leg, no skin, 75g (cooked weight) wholegrain rice, 50g sweetcorn, 50g carrots
- 75g any lean roast meat, thin gravy, 3 medium chunks roast potato, 50g peas, 25g scoop vanilla ice cream
- 1 can slimmer's soup, any flavour, 150g trout or herring, grilled, 2 small boiled potatoes, 50g carrots, 1 carton low-fat fruit yoghurt

TREATS (100 calories) Choose two each day.
• 1 small digestive biscuit
• 2 crispbreads with a little low-fat spread and sliced
  tomatoes
• 1 small banana

WEEKENDS

As for weekdays, but, after the first week, add 300
calories worth of chocolates daily from the list on page
213, OR 300 calories worth of recipes from Chapter 9.
You may also have one of the following each day:
• 1 glass dry wine
• 2 pub-measure 'short' drinks with low-calorie mixers
• $1/2$ pint beer or lager

EATING OUT

Choose clear soup or melon, then a simple fish or
meat dish, with vegetables and salads. At Indian
restaurants go for chicken tikka or tandoori, cucumber
riata, poppadam and plain boiled rice. At Italian
restaurants choose fish, cooked simply without sauces.
Carvery choices should be turkey with fresh vegetables

and a small ice cream to follow.

Diet for Sugar Addicts

Please note: it is possible that you will need additional counselling and help with your slimming campaign. Do have a check up with your doctor and also consult the list of eating disorders counselling services on page 235. If in doubt, do write to me at the address on page 235.

DAILY ALLOWANCES ^{1}/2 pint (275ml) skimmed milk for your tea and coffee, unlimited water and mineral water. Try to limit cups of tea and coffee to two a day, and try to drink herb tea instead. Drink lots of water.

FREE VEGETABLES Eat as much as you like from the 'free' vegetable list (page 86). Boil or steam vegetables, or serve them raw as salads. Do not add butter or oil. Instead, make your own dressing with lemon juice, vinegar, herbs and garlic.

CHOCOLATE After the first week, you may have 200 calories of chocolate every day (see list on page 213 or the recipes in Chapter 9). Eat it slowly and enjoy it.

• Do not add salt in cooking or sprinkle it on food.

STRATEGY

1. Take up yoga or meditation to help you cope. There are a number of good classes to go to — enquire locally.

2. Walk briskly for 20 minutes each day to help beat stress and rev up your metabolism. Even if you are in the kind of job where you use up a lot of energy rushing around, it is still important to walk. You may think you are 'on the go' all day long, but you are in fact getting little *real* exercise.

3. Make sure you eat regularly. The diet gives you four meals a day, plus treats. Spread them out, so your

blood sugar level is kept high. Missing meals is dangerous, both for your health and your slimming campaign.

4. Keep fresh fruit with you at all times to nibble when you feel low or tired.

5. Take a multi-vitamin capsule every day. Before a period, women can include Vitamin B6 and Evening Primrose Oil capsules.

6. When you have time off work get plenty of fresh air — walk, play tennis, swim.

7. Make a list of all the places you usually buy chocolates, and avoid them. Buy your chocolate allowance from somewhere different and get it every day, not in huge quantities.

WEEK ONE

EVERY DAY Eat *one* Breakfast, *two* Light Meals, *one*

Main Meal and *one* Treat.

BREAKFASTS (250 calories)

- 1 slice melon, 1 slice wholemeal toast topped with 2 tbsp cottage cheese, 1 medium banana
- 25g any unsweetened cereal, milk from allowance, 1 medium banana, small glass fruit juice
- 1 carton natural yoghurt with chopped apple and a sprinkling of nuts
- 2 crispbreads topped with 3 tsp peanut butter and sliced tomatoes, small glass fruit juice
- 1 sandwich of 2 slices bread, tomatoes, 12g grated Edam cheese

LIGHT MEALS (250 calories each)

Jacket potatoes Cook a 150g jacket potato and serve with salad and one of the following:

- 50g chopped ham or chicken
- 4 tbsp baked beans
- 1 carton low-calorie coleslaw

Meals on toast Top 1 slice wholemeal toast with one of the following, and add a large mixed salad and 1 apple

or pear:
- 50g sardines, drained of oil
- 1 small (125g) tin baked beans
- 1 grilled fish cake
- 1 size 3 egg, poached

Salads Make a huge mixed salad from the 'free' vegetable list (page 86) and add one of these accompaniments and 1 apple or pear:
- 50g cold chicken (no skin), 2 tbsp sweetcorn, 1 apple or orange
- 1 sliced size 3 egg, 1 crusty wholemeal roll
- 100g grilled fish, 1 slice wholemeal bread
- 50g corned beef, 1 medium banana

Sandwiches 2 slices wholemeal bread, salad from the 'free' list (page 86) and one of the following and 1 apple or orange:
- 2 tbsp cottage cheese
- 1 small chopped banana
- 50g tuna-in-brine

MAIN MEALS (400 calories)

Add plenty of 'free' vegetables (page 86) and salads.

- Any supermarket ready-meal of 400 calories or less
- 125g lean lamb chop, 215g can wholewheat spaghetti topped with sliced tomato, 25g grated Edam cheese, small bunch grapes
- 1 large slice of melon, 50g canned sardines on 1 slice toast, grilled tomatoes, watercress, 1 orange
- 150g grilled herring or tinned pilchards, 2 small boiled potatoes, 1 serving low-fat mousse
- 1 well-grilled beefburger, 2 tbsp sweetcorn, 150g jacket potato, 100g strawberries or raspberries
- 100g grilled liver, thin gravy, with 2 tbsp fresh orange juice added, 2 boiled potatoes, 2 tbsp sweetcorn or peas, 1 apple
- 200g chicken leg, no skin, grilled or roast with 150g jacket potato topped with 2 tbsp cottage cheese
- 200g any grilled white fish, 75g potatoes mashed with skimmed milk from allowance, 2 tbsp sweetcorn or carrots, 1 apple or orange

TREATS (100 calories) Choose one each day

- $1/2$ pint beer or lager
- 1 glass dry wine
- 2 pub-measure 'short' drinks with low-calorie mixers
- 1 large digestive biscuit
- 2 crispbreads topped with cottage cheese and sliced tomato
- 1 medium banana

WEEK TWO and subsequent weeks

Add 200 calories of chocolate (*see* list on page 213), OR 200 calories of desserts or drinks from the recipes on pages 173-206.

7

Massage, Meditation and Exercise

While you are following your Chocolate Diet, it is a good idea to increase the amount of exercise you take and to try out some do-it-yourself massage and meditation techniques.

Massage

A long, delicious massage with essential oils has almost the same naughty, self-indulgent feeling as working your way through a box of Black Magic, with none of the calories! Moreover, chocolate cravings could be forestalled by a quick massage at the appropriate time. Tension often leads to irritability and tiredness which, in turn, can lead to a chocolate binge. So, dealing with tension by soothing away those aches and pains is obviously a good idea. Here are some techniques for you to try both at work and home:

At Work   If you've had a really terrible day and the tea-time trolley (laden with chocolate bars, naturally) is about to appear, take time for a five-minute massage instead. If the boss objects, point out that Japanese workers usually have a masseuse on the staff.

1. Sit comfortably, with your bottom well back in your seat, feet apart and flat on the ground. If possible, place a small cushion in the hollow of your back. Now slowly raise your shoulders and drop them a few times, then circle your shoulders forwards and backwards, singly then together.

2. Now, place your right hand on your left shoulder and squeeze the tops of your shoulders with your fingers. Repeat with your left hand on your right shoulder.

3. Place the tips of your fingers on the back of your neck and, gently, massage each side of your vertebrae with your fingertips, stretching as far down your back as possible.

4. Place your thumbs under the back of your skull and spread your fingers out over your head. Press gently with your thumbs while rotating the balls of your fingers.

5. Place the tips of your middle fingers against the hollow each side of your brow-bone. Press gently, count six and relax.

6. Now move the same fingers to the top of your nose, placing them in the right-angled hollow made by your nose and brow-bone. Press upwards gently for a count of six, then relax.

(Nos. 5 and 6 are based on Japanese Shiatsu massage and are excellent for beating tension headaches and eyestrain.)

At home   You do not need a partner for this massage routine because all the movements can be performed by you. Try it when you are feeling low, or a bit lonely. Chocoholics who pig-out when partners are away working in the evening could devote a little time to this massage and then curl up with a good book — not a box of chocs.

You will need some oils for the routine. It is easy to buy essential oils these days but they can be expensive. The best plan is to buy a large bottle of cheap massage oil (or use ordinary cooking oil) and add just a few drops of essential oil to the base.

If you are feeling particularly stressed, tense and anxious choose one of the following oils, or a combination of three: bergamot, geranium, lavender, camomile, ylang-ylang, neroli, rose and geranium. If you are very tired and want to be perked up (perhaps your partner is due home later), try rosemary or bergamot. If your sex life needs livening up, go for sandalwood, jasmine or patchouli.

You will also need a warm room with sufficient space to lie down, a towel, massage oil with appropriate essential oils added, and tissues.

1. Lie on your back and relax for a minute. Pour a little oil on your tummy and rub it in with circular movements.

2. Roll over. Press your fingertips on either side of your spine and rub gently. Bring your hands above shoulder level and rub your shoulder blades, neck and shoulders with gentle stroking movements.

3. Sit up slowly, take some more lotion and knead and press your legs. Work from the thighs towards the knees, then back again. Now do the same thing down to your ankles and back again.

4. Still sitting, press the tips of your thumbs either side of your spine. Press for a few seconds, relax and

move your thumbs up about an inch (2.5cm). Repeat, working up as far as you can.

5. Stand up and knead and pinch your buttocks, then smooth on more oil in circular movements.

6. Now cover a chair with your towel and work some oil into your feet. The easiest way to do this is to rest one foot on the opposite thigh (like a modified 'half lotus' yoga position), and work really hard with fingers and thumbs all over the sole of your foot and between your toes. Repeat with the other foot.

7. Blot off the surplus oil with tissues, put on a bathrobe and rest on the bed for as long as you can. Set the alarm if you have an appointment as you may find that you drop off to sleep.

Meditation

Although there is no evidence that meditation alone will cure chocoholism, it can definitely help you to control your life which, in turn, can only make it easier to kick the habit. It provides a valuable pause in the day when you can clear problems out of your mind and switch off completely. Afterwards, you feel refreshed and more able to cope. You do not have to meditate sitting on a carpet dressed in a loin cloth. On the contrary, you can do it anywhere. Try this simple routine at work or at home:

1. Take your shoes off. Now loosen any constricting clothes, particularly around your waist. Undo those overtight jeans, unzip that too-tight skirt. Close your eyes and sit comfortably with your hands in your lap or on your knees.

2. Breathe in and out slowly and gently. Now notice the contact of your body on the chair and your feet

on the floor. Take a few comfortable breaths, imagining that you are taking in feelings of peace and tranquillity and breathing out all the stresses and tensions and worries of the day.

3. Concentrate on your feet and make them relax, then work right up your body, concentrating on each bit and 'telling' it to relax completely. When you are perfectly relaxed, take a few deep, satisfying breaths and enjoy the gentle rhythm and flow of your own breathing. You will almost feel as though you are weightless and floating.

4. After a minute or two, bring your body back to life. First, be aware of the contact between your body and the chair, your feet and the floor. Next, bring your toes back to life by wiggling them. Stretch out your legs. Wiggle your fingers, stretch your arms and hands. Give your whole body a really good stretch. Slowly open your eyes. You'll feel terrific.

Exercise

Here are three different sets of exercises which can all be beneficial for chocoholics. The first is based on yoga, the ancient routine which really does help you revitalise your body and mind as well as unwind and relax. The second is a stretching routine, which will sort out all the aches and creaks of the day which could set you reaching for chocs. The third is a more energetic programme of movements which can be performed at home. This is designed to rev up your metabolism and should only be followed if you are less than 3 stone overweight and fairly fit. So do be sensible. If you have doubts about your ability to do any of the movements, check with your doctor.

1. YOGA
'Hatha' or physical yoga is a series of ancient postures or positions that move and improve almost every part of the human body. Do each movement very slowly, aiming for your best possible posture.

The Corpse   This sounds deathly but it is a useful posture of deep relaxation which you should repeat before and after these exercises.

Lie on your back, legs apart, with feet flopping open. Your arms should be a little way away from your body, palms up, with fingers loosely curled. Now breathe deeply and evenly for one minute.

The Cobra   This is great for relieving tiredness and back pain and also helps sort out constipation and wind.

Lie face down with your legs together, chin on the floor.

Place your forearms on the floor, elbows close to your body, hands by your shoulders. Lift your head, arch your back and pull your shoulders back and down. Look at the ceiling. Hold the position for a count of six, then bend your arms slowly and lower your body to the starting position. You should breathe out as you raise your body, breathe in as you lower it. Repeat four times.

The Cat If you have ever seen a cat stretch, you will understand why our feline friends are so supple. This exercise will strengthen your spine and tone up your tummy.

Go down on your hands and knees with your hands directly underneath your shoulders, fingers facing forwards. Slowly, let your back sink down, pushing your bottom up and out. Look up at the ceiling. Slowly, reverse the position by arching your back and pulling in your tummy. Drop your chin on to your chest. Hold for a count of five and repeat, then sit back on your heels for a few moments.

The Coil If you have a wobbly bottom, this exercise is excellent. It tones the buttock muscles brilliantly. It also increases strength and mobility in the neck and helps flatten your tummy.

Lie on your back with your legs and feet together, toes pointed, and palms of your hands pressing downwards on the floor. Now bend your knees and bring them in as close to your chest as you can manage. Interlock your fingers and loop your hands over your knees. Pull your knees with your hands and raise your head towards them. Hold for a count of five, then lower your head to the floor and relax. Repeat twice and stretch out in the Corpse position (see page 138), for just a few seconds.

Salute to the Sun   This is a series of 12 movements which give a complete, all-round exercise in a very short time. It is ideal for early morning and really does set you up for the day. Try it once you have mastered the four basic exercises above.

The alternate stretching and bending helps improve circulation and aids breathing. Your digestion, tummy, back, arm and leg muscles are also given a boost. It is best to do this standing in loose clothes with bare feet on a soft rug. Try it once, then repeat if you have time:

1. Stand with your back straight, feet together. Press the palms of your hands together in front of your chest, with forearms horizontal and shoulders relaxed.

2. Now inhale, raising your arms above your head. Stretch upwards looking at the ceiling, tighten your buttocks and lean backwards, keeping your head and arms in a straight line.

3. Bend forward from your hips, exhaling as you do so. Tuck your head down to touch your knees and let your hands touch your legs. Now bend your knees so the palms of your hands touch the floor.

4. Look up, and take your left leg back as far as possible, with your knee on the floor. Your right knee should be bent, right heel on the floor. Arch your back.

5. Keeping your weight on your arms and hands, stretch your right leg back beside your left, so your legs, body and head make a straight line.

6. Now bend your arms and place your forehead, chest and knees on the floor. Breathe out and pull in your tummy. Breathe normally and take a mid-exercise rest for a few moments.

7. Push down on your hands, straightening your arms and arch your spine, lower your shoulders and look up. You are now in the Cobra pose, described above.

8. Raise your bottom into the air, straightening your legs and arms and letting your head hang down between them.

9. Transfer your weight on to your legs, lowering your heels.

10. Bring your right foot forward, and place the sole on the floor. Lower your left knee, look up and inhale.

11. Bring your left foot forward next to the right one, straightening your legs, bend forward, clasp your legs and exhale.

12. Now 'uncoil', raising your arms, body, and stretching so your arms are above your head. Slowly, go back to position 1.

2. STRETCHING EXERCISES

Do you ever arrive home from work feeling tired, hunched, and with nagging indigestion that won't go away? Before you reach for a drink, some medication or a comforting chocolate, go upstairs to your bedroom and do some very simple stretching exercises. They can help you unwind, internally as well as externally. You will find that those aches and creaks disappear and you feel full of life. Amazingly those hunger pangs (which weren't really hunger pangs at all) will have vanished.

Total Stretch This is good for your back, legs, arms and tummy muscles and really does help you unwind. It is a great one to do if you've just driven home through congested traffic or arrived at your hotel after a long flight (leave the complementary chocolate on the pillow alone!).

Stand, feet together, arms above your head, fingers clasped loosely. Look up at your hands. Bend your knees and bring your hands down slowly to the horizontal position. Let your hands fall sideways and down, and relax your head forward. Pause, then reverse the movement. Repeat five times, breathing in as you raise your body, out as you lower it.

Leg and Arm Spine Stretch This is super for legs, arms, tummy and posture. It is the one you often see athletes doing before a race to help them warm up and prevent injury.

Stand straight, feet together, hands by your sides. Now take your left foot back, keeping your weight forward, left heel off the ground. Raise your right arm above your head. Raise your left leg and push your right arm back, keeping your right leg straight. Repeat five times with your left leg, right arm, then five times with your right arm, left leg.

Thigh and Hip Stretch If you have been sitting down in a train or bus, or at work all day, this will help to sort out that cramped feeling in your bottom. It will also help slim your hips and thighs.

Sit on the floor, hands behind you for support, back straight, knees bent. Now swing your hips to the left, lowering both knees to touch the floor. Repeat to the right. Repeat the complete movement, right and left, five times.

Side and Waist Stretch By improving your posture, you can appear much taller and slimmer. This exercise helps to whittle inches off your waistline and midriff and encourages you to sit and stand straight.

Stand with your feet about 2 feet (60cm) apart, hands by your sides. Now raise your right arm above your head, and bend your body, from the waist only, over to the left as far as you can go. Straighten up and repeat to the right. Repeat five times each side. After this mini work-out, you should be ready to tackle anything!

3. ENERGETIC EXERCISES

This routine is designed as a three-times-weekly work-out which will help rev up your metabolism. It is only suitable for slimmers who have 3 stone or less to lose and are reasonably fit. Do not attempt it if you are in bad shape. If in doubt, check with your doctor. Some lively music will help you stay the course!

Warm-up   Start the routine by doing the Stretching Exercises above, repeating the Total Stretch exercise again at the end of the set.

Bent-Knee Sit Ups   This is an excellent tummy-toner and the bent-knee position helps prevent back strain.

Lie on your back on the floor, with your feet on the floor, knees bent and legs slightly apart. Raise your arms to knee level, hands together, fingers straight. Leading with your head 'roll up' your back as far as you can to a sitting position, arms thrusting through your legs. Slowly, roll down, head last, until you are in the starting position. Repeat five to ten times, increasing repetitions as you improve.

Bottom and Hip Tightener If you hate your bottom. this is a superb exercise for you. But carry on dieting, too!

Kneel on the floor, placing your hands on the floor in front of you at shoulder level. Stretch your right leg out to one side, with the foot pointing forwards. Now raise the leg as high as you can keeping it at right angles to your body. Lower, repeat five times, then five times with the other leg. (To make this exercise slightly harder, and increase the work for your buttock and thigh muscles, do it with your knee bent, for the same number of repetitions.)

Thigh Lunge This is a controlled exercise which is harder than it sounds, but does great things for your thighs. Try not to wobble!

Stand with both feet on the floor, hands on your hips, with your right leg straight out in front, left leg behind, feet wide apart. Distribute your weight evenly between your feet. Now bend your right leg, moving your weight on to it. Keep your back straight and go down as low as you can without bending forward. Bend and straighten ten times. Swap legs and repeat.

Waist, Spine and Tummy Toner   There are two separate movements in this exercise. It is fun and makes you feel very lively.

Stand with your feet apart, hands clasped above your head. Turn your body to the left, then lean forward from the waist, head down, arms straight out. Keep your head and arms in a straight line, and circle the upper part of your body down then up again, alternate ways. Repeat five times.

Now, lean forwards from the waist and thrust your hands through your legs, palms down, as far as is comfortably possible. Raise your body, place your hands on your waistline and lean back. Repeat five times.

Step Ups   This is the original version of the popular 'stepping' routines which are popular in health clubs and gyms. It is great for building up stamina.

Stand facing a small bench or the bottom step of the stairs. Now step up on to the bench with your left foot, bring your right foot up to meet it, then step down with your right foot, and bring your left foot down to meet it. Make sure you keep your back straight, your hands by your sides.

Running on the Spot   End your work-out with an 'indoor jog'. Run on the spot, with your back straight and your elbows bent. Do 50 paces, then relax.

8

How to Stay Slim and Eat Chocolate

So, you have reached your 'goal' weight and are wondering if you will be strong enough to stay in shape for good. This is the most important moment of your life. For, as every slimmer knows, it is far harder to keep weight off than to lose it in the first place.

This is particularly true for chocoholics, who are exposed to their greatest temptation every single day.

Don't worry. I promise you that you can stay slim and enjoy a certain amount of chocolate without 'pigging-out' if you use the strategy outlined in this chapter.

Face up to Your Success

The hardest task you face right now is to enjoy your achievement. Yes, amazing though it may seem, many slimmers find that reaching their target weight brings along a whole set of problems which they find difficult to cope with. Here are six examples, and how to tackle them:

1. *Coping with relationships*   Your family or partner may feel threatened by the 'new' you. Suddenly, you are slim, dynamic and attractive, no longer plagued by the ups and downs of temperament that invariably accompany chocoholism. They are rattled, and may express this worry negatively, by being unreasonable, unhelpful or unloving. What you should do: be extra attentive but be firm in your

determination to look good and do what you want to do. They will soon adapt to the new you once they realise that the old you is still intact, too.

2. *Tackling challenges*   When you were overweight it was very easy to use this as an excuse for opting out. You had a great reason for avoiding social events, work opportunities, sport, anything which might involve making an effort. Now, you no longer have that excuse. What you should do: dip one toe in the water at a time! Go to that party, book up that holiday, apply for that job — but don't do all three at once. Instead, revel in your new body by making the very best of your appearance. Invest in some new clothes, a good haircut, a night out. As soon as you realise that challenges are fun you will start to enjoy them instead of fearing them.

3. *Enjoying sex*   For many chocoholics (especially Comfort Eaters and Romantics), chocs take the place of sex. Once your body is in great shape, there is no longer any reason for avoiding one of life's

greatest pleasures. It is at this moment that you may realise that the sex-life you so carefully avoided wasn't all that great in the first place. Or you may suddenly discover that there is no one to share your new-found sex-drive! What you should do: where there is an existing relationship which has gone sour, it is well worth trying to improve things. Your partner may be, quite rightly, fed up with your attitude and reluctant to get things going again. Some gentle wooing, romantic nights out and sexy underwear will work wonders. If not, counselling may be the answer. If you have avoided meeting the opposite sex and have no partner, it's a good idea to start being social again. Don't rush into a sexual relationship, though, until you have enjoyed some good old-fashioned romance first.

4. *Wish fulfilment*   Many slimmers believe, erroneously, that being slim will make all their wildest dreams come true. Their partner will suddenly love them more, all their money worries will disappear, and they will suddenly enjoy a Hollywood lifestyle.

Sorry, but life isn't like that. True, being slim makes you feel better about yourself and more able to cope but it doesn't automatically make life rosier. Face this important fact head on and you will not be disappointed (and you will not reach for a box of chocs to cheer you up!).

5. *Size and power*   Some overweight people subconsciously enjoy the power that being fat brings. They like to be noticed and talked about. Men, particularly, are inclined to equate size with potency: the theory being that if their beer-belly is big it does not matter about other parts of their anatomy. If you suddenly miss being large, remember that fitness is macho too. You can always build up some muscle by working out.

6. *Dealing with jealousy*   At first, it is lovely to be congratulated on your weight loss, but after a time you may realise that one or two of your closest friends are jealous of your success. They start making digs about your 'sunken cheeks' and 'thin

legs', and follow up by dragging you into cafés for slices of chocolate cake and gateau. Be strong. Recognise this as a sign of their insecurity, not yours. Deal with it by politely refusing their tempting offers You *can* do it.

7. *Setting new targets*   When you reach 'goal' there is always a moment of deflation because you no longer have the challenge ahead of hitting your target. Well, set another target — but this time make it to do with your home, work or fitness. Happiness is all about tackling new things and stretching yourself, so go for it!

How to Stay in Control

There are ten important rules you must follow if you want to stay slim:

1. *Eat regularly*   You must follow a sensible eating plan such as the one in this chapter if you are to keep

your chocoholism under control. That means having a meal or snack every few hours throughout the day. Do not ever let your blood sugar level get so low that you crave sweet foods.

2. *Be prepared*   Every week, think about the various tasks you have to do and the appointments you have made. Plan your eating programme as well as your working and social programme.

3. *Take food with you*   Never go anywhere without some fruit or a low-calorie snack in your shopping bag, briefcase or tool box. Don't be a sitting target for temptation.

4. *Keep busy*   Pack plenty of activity into your life, so food takes second, third, or even fourth place. Re-decorate, go on bus rides, join local societies.

5. *Exercise regularly*   Use the programme in Chapter Eight of this book to help you stay in amazing shape and rev up your metabolism.

6. *Have plenty of treats*   You deserve the best. Allow yourself the sheer luxury of a half-day off to walk in the park, visit a gallery, curl up with a good book or simply stay in bed with your partner.

7. *Enjoy your meals and your chocolate allowance*   You will see that your Maintenance Diet allows you plenty of food, including a generous ration of chocolate and choccy dishes. Please eat them up and enjoy them.

8. *Keep your body image strong*   Every day, look at yourself in the mirror and make a point of enjoying what you see. Vanity is healthy. Take time out to visualise yourself in future situations like a family party, wedding or holiday, looking fit, well, and slim. Imagine every detail, from what you are wearing, to the food you are eating and the company you are in.

9. *Relax*   Stress is a diet killer. Beat it by taking short, inexpensive breaks whenever possible. Psychologists

say that they are better for you than a longer holiday which can be stressful in itself.

10. *Weigh yourself weekly*   It is crazy to weigh in more often than that because fluid changes in the body can play havoc with your 'official' weight. Instead, step on the scales once a week, at the same time of day, wearing the same clothes. Allow yourself a 5lb 'ceiling' above your goal weight. If you go above that level, go back on your Chocolate Diet for a week or so. Even if you slip back, don't panic. Slimming may be a lifetime's occupation, but it is fun, too.

Choes around the World

Once you have managed to lose weight and control your chocoholism, you can start enjoying it. The best way to eat chocolate is in small amounts, savouring every little bit. It is easier to eat less when you pay more, so indulge yourself with expensive chocolate once in a while. Here is a guide to some of the best places to buy 'posh' chocolate:

London, England   Leonidas, the famous Belgian chocolatiers, have a shop on the ground floor at Selfridges with a selection of delicious hand-made luxury chocs. Charbonnet and Walker in Bond Street is the shop for the real connoisseur but don't visit it if you are strapped for cash. Any branch of Thornton's is choc-full of goodies!

Paris, France   Try Maisons du Chocolat for amazing centres, incredible truffles and gorgeous slab chocolate.

Geneva, Switzerland   Jenny's at the railway station is the best shop but amazing chocs are everywhere.

Zurich, Switzerland   Sprungli or Teuscher sell the sensational Pfister chocolates — every mouthful is orgasmic!

Brussels, Belgium   Any branch of Leonidas or Godiva is a chocoholic's paradise.

Aspen, USA   At the Rocky Mountain Chocolate Factory the chocolate is made right in the shop window, so it is almost impossible not to go in and taste it. They sell huge slabs but it is much safer to buy the smaller bars.

Hong Kong   If you stay at the Hilton, try the Gerard Dubois chocs — lovely.

Copenhagen, Denmark   Try the help-yourself chocolate bar at the Airport but do eat a protein-packed snack first.

Hamburg, Germany   Go to the Condi Café in the Vier Jahreszeitsen, where they make their own, yummy chocs.

Vienna, Austria   Look for the Kuvkonditorei Oberlaa branches where they sell chocolates made by master chocolatier, Karl Shuhmacher.

Best chocs by aeroplane Chocoholic travellers recommend the Lufthansa and Swiss Air selections, because their after-dinner chocolates are hand-made by small manufacturers.

Your Maintenance Diet

Here is the diet which will help you stay slim. It allows about 2,000 calories for women, and 2,500 for men. Follow it for two weeks after you reach your target weight. If you are still losing, increase your calories by 100 each week, choosing items from the list at the end of this chapter (sorry, this does not include chocolate) until you maintain a steady weight.

Women can also have 150 calories daily of chocolate (including bars, sweets, individual chocs, biscuits or dishes chosen from the recipes in Chapter 9), men can have 200 calories. This can be eaten in two or three 'lumps' during the week but not all at one go. Avoid buying it all at once, and make sure you really enjoy every mouthful.

In France, chocolate connoisseurs (mostly very slim people!) like to take their daily treat of dark, delicious, expensive chocolate with a glass of wine or cognac. Since you are allowed a daily alcohol ration, there is no reason why you shouldn't do the same. One of the successful chocoholic slimmers who tried my diet now has a very expensive chocolate wafer mint in bed every night, plus a small brandy while she watches an erotic video. This is on the nights when her husband is away working. When he's home, they only manage to watch about 20 minutes of the video!

DAILY ALLOWANCES

You may have $^1/2$ pint (275ml) semi-skimmed milk for your tea and coffee, plus unlimited water and mineral water. (Go easy on the caffeine, and try to include more water and herbal drinks in your diet. Camomile, lemon and tropical fruit teas are all delicious.) Although diet soft drinks contain very few calories and most eating programmes allow them, do take it easy. Unfortunately, too many of these sweet-tasting drinks could have a nasty effect on your taste-buds and turn you into a chocolate junkie again. Beware!

You can also have unlimited vegetables from the list on page 86. Serve them imaginatively, as salads with lemon juice, herbs and vinegar dressings, or lightly boiled, steamed or stir fried in very little oil. Pile them up on your plate at every meal so you never feel deprived.

MALE EXTRAS   Choose *two* each day.
• 2 large slices of wholemeal bread with a little low-fat spread
• 1 pint beer or lager
• 120g mashed potato made with skimmed milk
• 50g any lean meat

ALCOHOL ALLOWANCE   Choose *one* each day.
• $1/2$ pint beer or lager
• 1 glass dry wine
• 2 pub-measure 'short' drinks with low-calorie mixers only

Non-drinkers can have an extra slice of bread or a small wholemeal roll.

EVERY DAY Eat *one* Breakfast, *one* Light Meal, *one* Supper and *one* Metabolic Boosting High Protein Snack which you should eat when you feel that your energy is flagging and your taste-buds are tingling.

BREAKFASTS

- 2 rashers well-grilled back bacon, grilled tomatoes, 1 slice wholemeal toast, 1 apple
- Sandwich of 2 slices wholemeal bread with one of these fillings:
    - 1 medium banana
    - 2 rashers well-grilled streaky bacon and tomatoes
    - 50g grated low-fat Cheddar cheese
- 50g any unsweetened cereal, with milk from allowance, 1 size 3 egg, 2 crispbreads with a little low-fat spread
- 1 carton low-fat yoghurt, any flavour, 1 slice wholemeal toast topped with a little Marmite or 1 tsp jam or marmalade, 100ml unsweetened fruit juice
- Breakfast milkshake made by blending together 125ml semi-skimmed milk (extra to allowance), 1 large chopped banana, 1 carton low-calorie banana

yoghurt, sprinkling of cocoa powder

LIGHT MEALS

Jacket Potatoes   250g jacket potato with salad and vegetables from 'free' list and one of these fillings:

• 4 tbsp baked beans and 12g grated Edam cheese

• 1 carton low-calorie coleslaw

• 2 tbsp natural yoghurt mixed with a little horseradish sauce and 50g chopped chicken or ham (no skin or fat)

• 1 small can tuna-in-brine, mashed with lemon juice

OR Choose your Jacket Potato meal from a takeaway such as Spud-U-Like where you may choose any of these fillings: baked beans, cottage cheese with chives, Mexican Bean salad, Spring Salad or Sweetcorn.

Meals on Toast   2 slices wholemeal toast topped with one of the following plus 1 apple, orange, pear or small banana:

• 1 poached egg and 4 tbsp baked beans or canned spaghetti in tomato sauce

• 1 can tuna-in-in brine topped with 25g grated Edam

cheese
- grilled tomatoes topped with 2 rashers well-grilled back bacon
- 50g mushrooms poached in chicken stock, mixed with 50g lean chopped ham

Meals with a Chocolate Recipe
- 250g chicken leg, no skin, huge mixed salad. 1 portion Chocolate Banana Cake (*see* recipe, page 180)
- Chocolate Banana Sandwich (*see* recipe, page 203), 1 apple
- 150g any grilled fish, grilled tomatoes and salad from the 'free' list, Chocolate Mousse (*see* recipe, page 193), 1 apple, a few grapes

Salads   Large mixed salad from 'free' list with lemon juice or vinegar and herb dressing with one of the following:
- 250g chicken wing, skin removed, 1 small wholemeal roll with a little low-fat spread, 1 large banana or 2 apples or pears

- Medium piece quiche (cheese, meat or fish), 1 apple, orange, or small banana or low-calorie yoghurt
- 150g smoked fish, 1 slice wholemeal bread with a little low-fat spread, slice of lemon, a few grapes

Sandwiches   2 slices wholemeal bread with salad from 'free' list and one of these fillings and accompaniments:
- 50g chicken, ham or any lean meat without fat or skin, 1 apple, pear or small banana

MAIN MEALS
Cold Meals   Large mixed salad from the 'free' list with one of the following:
- 50g any cold, lean meat, 1 wholemeal roll with a little low-fat spread, 25g Edam or low-fat hard cheese
- 1 medium slice quiche, 2 tbsp sweetcorn, 1 apple
- Any supermarket ready-meal under 400 calories, 1 slice wholemeal bread with a little low-fat spread, 1 banana

Hot Meals
- 75g pasta (dry weight) topped with one of the

following:

- tinned tomatoes with 100g shelled prawns, garlic, herbs, large mixed salad; 25g scoop vanilla icecream with 1 portion Chocolate Sauce (*see* recipe, page 201) *OR* 1 small wholemeal roll with 12g Camembert or other soft cheese
- 125g lean lamb or pork chop, grilled, thin gravy, large portion 'free' vegetables, 75g mashed potato (use skimmed milk from allowance for mashing), baked apple with 1 tbsp yoghurt
- 125g lean rump or fillet steak, grilled, 75g oven chips, grilled tomatoes, watercress, large mixed salad and vegetables from the 'free' list
- 1 large slice of melon or ½ grapefruit with ginger and/or artificial sweetener, 100g gammon steak, grilled, 2 tbsp peas, 1 slice pineapple, canned in juice, 150g jacket potato, large portion salad and 'free' vegetables
- 100g calves' liver, grilled, 1 rasher well-grilled back bacon, grilled tomatoes, vegetables from the 'free' list, 1 portion Chocolate and Raisin Rice Pudding

(*see* recipe, page 198) or Chocolate Coconut Icecream (*see* recipe, page 188)

- Casserole of 100g lean stewing beef cooked in 1 can low-calorie tomato soup with sliced onions, 2 tbsp sliced carrots, herbs, garlic and beef stock, vegetables from the 'free' list, 1 large banana

Vegetarian Meals

- 2 vegetable burgers, grilled, grilled tomatoes, 75g oven chips, large mixed salad from the 'free' list, 2 tbsp peas, 25g scoop vanilla ice cream with 1 portion Chocolate Sauce (*see* recipe, page 201)
- Any supermarket veggie ready-meal under 400 calories with additional vegetables and salad from the 'free' list and 12g grated low-fat Cheddar cheese

Eating out

Choose melon or clear soup as a starter and then go for lean meat or fish (no sauces) and a good selection of vegetables. At Indian restaurants, choose Chicken Tikka or Tandoori with plain boiled rice and salad. Chinese restaurants are more difficult. Your best bet is a Chicken Chop Suey with plain boiled rice. Avoid all fatty foods, those with creamy sauces, and the sweet trolley unless you are feeling very strong indeed. If you do go 'over the top', make up for it by cutting out your alcohol and chocolate allowance for a couple of days.

Metabolic Boosting High Protein Snacks

Choose one each day. Make sure you have your snack with you – most of these are easy to pack:

- 2 crispbreads with scraping of Marmite and 1 small carton cottage cheese
- 2 sticks celery, filled with 1 heaped dsp peanut butter
- 50g thin ham, spread with 25g Philadelphia Light spread, rolled up and cut into bite-sized pieces
- 3 Matthews Mini Kievs with grilled tomatoes
- 25g Edam cheese on a skewer with chopped green peppers, tomatoes, mushrooms, 2 crispbreads with scraping of low-fat spread
- 1 slice low-calorie bread, 1 cold fish finger and salad
- 50g John West prawns, drained, 75g boiled rice, onion, 1 tsp peas, 1 tsp diced carrot

- 1 mug Batchelors Slim a Soup Special Tomato and Vegetable with Croutons topped with 12g grated low-fat Cheddar
- 25g Edam cheese, 1 apple

100-CALORIE EXTRAS (If you are still losing weight 2 weeks after reaching your target weight add one of these each day for a week. If you are still losing add another, and so on.)

- 1 slice wholemeal bread or small wholemeal roll with a little low-fat spread
- 75g potato, mashed with skimmed milk
- 75g any pasta (dry weight)
- 50g chicken (no skin) or lean ham
- 1 large banana or 2 medium apples, oranges or pears
- 2 tbsp sweetcorn and 3 tbsp peas or carrots
- 1 low-fat pork sausage

9

Choc Full of Taste!

*H*ere is a selection of choccy recipes which have been cut down to the minimum calories, especially for chocoholics. You may include them in your diet as part of your daily chocolate calorie allowance only. For instance, if you are on one of the programmes that allows 200 calories of chocolate each day, you can either choose that from the chocolate list (page 213) *or* from the recipes given here. Not both, sorry!

Don't forget, these dishes are to enjoy. Don't feel guilty about savouring every single mouthful. A word of warning: if you are cooking up something just for yourself and the ingredients are given for four people, you could be in trouble. It is safer to divide the ingredients into four and make just one portion, invite three hungry people around to share the meal, or make up four portions and hide three in the fridge or a cake tin with a lid! For biscuit recipes, it is essential to store the goodies in a tin or make them only for special occasions when you are expecting a horde of hungry guests. No cheating, please!

Aphroidisiac Dishes

These are mouthwatering, fun-shaped treats for lovers. Don't forget, the more real love and affection you have, the less likely you are to be zapped by the 'false' kind, conjured up by the phenylethylamine in chocolate.

Use these recipes to seduce the important person, or people, in your life and yourself (and don't forget to count the calories as part of your daily chocolate allowance)!

CHOCOLATE ALMOND NIBBLES

50g self-raising flour

$1/4$ level tsp (2.5 ml) baking powder

25g cocoa powder

25g almonds, blanched and chopped

150g soft brown sugar

orange rind of $1/2$ orange

50g butter

75g low-fat soft cheese

2 large eggs

1. Sieve together the flour, baking powder and cocoa.
2. Add the almonds, sugar and orange rind. Beat the butter and cheese together.
3. Beat into the dry ingredients and then add the eggs, mixing thoroughly.
4. Spoon into a greased 7-inch (18cm) cake tin and level the top. Bake for 50 minutes at 160°C, 325°F, Gas 3, until cooked.
5. Cool on a wire rack, and cut into 16 squares. Store them out of sight in a tin until needed.

Makes 16 pieces *80 calories per piece*

CHOUX BOOBS
Pastry 1/4 pint (150ml) water
50g low-fat spread for cooking
70g plain flour, sieved
pinch of salt
2 large eggs, lightly beaten
Filling 16 level tbsp (240ml) chocolate icecream
8oz (25g) sliced strawberries or raspberries
Topping 8tsps (40ml) strawberry jam
8 chocolate buttons

1. Place water and spread in a small saucepan and bring to the boil over a moderate heat.

2. Remove from the heat and immediately add the sieved flour and salt. Beat with a wooden spoon until mixture leaves the sides of the pan. Cool slightly.

3. Beat the eggs in small quantities into the cooled mixture.

4. Place 8tbsp (120ml) of the mixture on a baking sheet lined with non-stick baking paper.

5. Bake near the top of a pre-heated oven 220°C, 425°F, Gas 7 for 20 minutes. Reduce the temperature to 190°C, 375°F, Gas 5 and cook for another 10 minutes.

6. Slit base of buns to allow steam to escape and then cool.

7. When cold, fill the buns with icecream and fruit.

8. Top with jam and a single chocolate button.

Serves 6 *160 calories per portion*

CHOC PEAKS

50g rolled oats

3tbsp (45ml) whisky

1tsp (5ml) clear honey

juice of 1 lemon

225g low-fat cottage cheese, sieved

150ml carton low-fat yoghurt, chilled

50g stoned dates, chopped

15g dark chocolate for decoration

1. Spread the oats on a baking tray and toast lightly under the grill.
2. Place the whisky, honey and lemon juice in a small bowl and stir.
3. Place the cottage cheese and yoghurt in a large bowl and gradually beat in the whisky mixture, dates and most of the oats.
4. Divide between four serving dishes and decorate with a few oats. Chill and sprinkle with grated chocolate just before serving.

Serves 4 *170 calories per portion*

CHOCOLATE WOBBLY BITS

(Microwave recipe)

2tbsp (30ml) cornflour

1tbsp (15ml) cocoa powder

1tbsp (15ml) Fructose

275ml skimmed milk

4tsp (1.25ml) vanilla essence

1tsp (5ml) low-fat spread

strips of orange to decorate

1. Blend cornflour, cocoa and Fructose together in a large jug.
2. Gradually stir in the milk.
3. Cook on maximum, uncovered, for 1 minute. Stir well and then cook on maximum for a further 30 seconds or until the mixture thickens.
3. Stir again, then add the low-fat spread and vanilla essence.
4. Pour into individual dishes, cover with clingfilm and leave to set.
5. Decorate with orange strips before serving.

Serves 2 *125 calories per portion*

Cakes and Biscuits

Once you have trained your palate to accept smaller quantities of chocolate, it is safe to indulge in these. A word of warning however: make your cakes and biscuits in small batches only and store them, out of sight, in an airtight container.

CHOCOLATE BANANA CAKE

15g cocoa
90g wholemeal self-raising flour
1 level tsp (5ml) baking powder
50g walnuts
100g margarine
5 level tbsp (75ml) Hermesetas Sprinkle Sweet
1 large ripe banana
2 eggs, size 2

1. Sieve together the cocoa, flour and baking powder.
2. Chop the walnuts.
3. Cream together the margarine and Sprinkle Sweet.

4. Mash the banana and beat into the creamed mixture.

5. Lightly beat the eggs and mix them into the creamed mixture a little at a time.

6. Stir in the flour mixture and walnuts.

7. Turn into a greased and lined 7-inch (18cm) square shallow tin. Bake in a preheated oven at 180°C, 350°F, Gas 4 for 30 minutes. Cool on a wire rack.

Makes 16 squares *110 calories per portion*

CHOC CHIP COOKIES

225g self-raising flour
pinch of salt
150g sunflower margarine
100g caster sugar
50g plain chocolate chips
1 egg, size 3, beaten

1. Sift the flour and add the salt. Rub in the margarine until the mixture resembles breadcrumbs.

2. Add the sugar and the chocolate chips.

3. Next add the egg and mix to a firm dough.

4. Knead gently on a floured surface until smooth.

5. Place inside a plastic bag and chill for 30 minutes.

6. Roll the dough out thinly and, using a 2-inch (5cm) cutter, cut out 30 biscuits.

7. Place on a lightly greased baking sheet and prick all over with a fork.

8. Bake for 12–15 minutes at 180°C, 350°F, Gas 4.

9. Allow to cool on a baking sheet.

Makes 30 biscuits *90 calories per cookie*

CAROB DISHES

Most chocoholics find it difficult to enjoy the taste of carob in 'pretend' chocolate bars. However, this well-known chocolate substitute is more palatable when used in cooking especially if it is combined with fruit. It also has the advantage of having none of the side-effects of chocolate, so the urge to eat more than is good for you is not so compelling.

It is worth trying these recipes. Carob is available from most health food shops.

CAROB BLACK FOREST GATEAU

3 eggs, size 3, separated

3oz (85g) caster sugar

70g plain white flour

15g carob powder

175g black cherries, canned in natural juice, stoned

150g Shape Double

1. Whisk the egg whites and sugar together until thick and foamy.
2. Mix the flour and carob powder together. Gently, fold into the whites, and pour into 2 loose-bottomed, lightly oiled and lined 8-inch (20cm) cake tins.
3. Bake at 180°C, 350°F, Gas 4 for 15–20 minutes until springy to the touch. Allow to cool on a wire rack.
4. Chop the cherries. Whisk the cream into soft peaks and fold into the fruit. Sandwich the sponge together with the mixture, reserving some to decorate the top.

Serves 8 *160 calories per portion*

CAROB MOUSSE

90g carob bar

grated rind and juice of $^1/_2$ small orange

2 eggs, size 2, separated

1 tsp (5ml) powdered gelatine

fine strips of orange rind, for decoration

1. Place the carob in a small bowl over a pan of simmering water and stir until melted.
2. Remove from heat and stir in the grated orange rind and beat in the egg yolks.
3. Place the orange juice in another small basin and sprinkle on the gelatine. Leave to stand for 5 minutes. Place the basin in a pan containing a little simmering water and leave until the gelatine has dissolved.
4. Stir into the carob mixture.
5. Whisk the egg whites to form stiff peaks and fold into the mixture.
6. Divide between 4 individual serving dishes. Chill in the refrigerator until set. Decorate with strips of orange rind.

Serves 4 *180 calories per portion*

ORANGE CAROB CAKE

75g low-fat cooking margarine

225g self-raising flour

4tbsp (60ml) Hermesetas Sprinkle Sweet

100g carob bar, chopped

grated rind and juice of 1 orange

a little skimmed milk

1 egg, size 3

1. Preheat the oven to 180°C, 350°F, Gas 4. Line and brush a 2lb loaf tin lightly with oil.
2. Rub the margarine into the flour in a mixing bowl.
3. Add the Sprinkle Sweet, orange rind and carob. Stir lightly.
4. Squeeze the orange and pour the juice into a measuring jug.
5. Add enough milk to make the liquid up to $1/4$ pint (150ml).
6. Beat the egg and pour into the dry ingredients. Add the orange juice and milk mixture, stir and turn into the loaf tin.
7. Bake for about 1 hour or until an inserted skewer

comes out clean. Cool, then turn out on a wire rack. Serve in slices.

Serves 6 *160 calories per portion*

Drinks

Here are some great recipes for long, delicious chocolate drinks. They are very tasty but not too high in calories. Sip them slowly, enjoying the full flavour of the chocolate and their scrumptious ingredients.

CARIBBEAN MILKSHAKE

1 pint (575ml) skimmed milk

2–3 level tsps (10–15ml) drinking chocolate

150g tub natural, low-fat yoghurt

1 banana, cut into three pieces

1 tbsp (15ml) rum (optional)

1 level tsp (5ml) chopped nuts to decorate

1. Place all the ingredients in a blender and mix until smooth.
2. Divide between 4 glasses and decorate with nuts.

Serves 4 *110 calories per glass*

CHOCOLATE MINT MILKSHAKE

272ml skimmed milk

1 tbsp (15ml) drinking chocolate powder

2–3 drops peppermint essence

3 ice cubes

Hermesetas Sprinkle Sweet to taste

1. Place all ingredients in a liquidiser and blend for 30 seconds.
2. Pour into a tall glass and drink slowly!

Serves 1 *130 calories per glass*

Frozen Desserts

Frozen desserts and ice cream are easy to make at home and safer for slimmers than the shop-bought kind because it is easier to control the calories. These are good for dinner parties or pure self-indulgence.

CHOCOLATE COCONUT ICE CREAM

150ml semi-skimmed milk

50g dessicated coconut

1 level tbsp (15ml) cocoa

2 level tbsp (30ml) Hermesetas Sprinkle Sweet

1 level tsp (5ml) gelatine

2 tbsp (30ml) water

150ml whipping cream

150ml half-fat evaporated milk

2 tbsp (30ml) Malibu

1. Place the milk, coconut and cocoa in a small pan and heat until boiling, stirring all the time.
2. Turn into a basin and stir in the Sprinkle Sweet.

3. Dissolve the gelatine in the water and add to the milk mixture. Leave until cold but not set.

4. Whip the cream until it forms soft peaks. Whip the evaporated milk until it is light and fluffy.

5. Fold the cream and evaporated milk into the milk mixture with the Malibu.

6. Turn into a plastic container and freeze for 2 hours.

7. Turn into a chilled bowl and whisk to break down the ice crystals. Return to the container and freeze until solid.

Serves 8 *160 calories per portion*

CHOCOLATE AND MINT ICE CREAM

150ml)natural low fat yoghurt

150g skimmed-milk soft cheese

peppermint flavouring

green food colouring (optional)

3tbsp (45ml) Hermesetas Sprinkle Sweet

2 egg whites

15g plain chocolate drops

1. Gradually beat the yoghurt into the cheese then whisk together until light.
2. Whisk in a few drops of peppermint flavouring, food colouring if desired, and the Hermesetas Sprinkle Sweet.
3. Spoon the mixture into a shallow metal container and cover. Place in the freezer and leave for one hour.
4. Empty into a chilled bowl and whisk using a mixer to break down the ice crystals.
5. Freeze for another 30 minutes and repeat the whisking process.
6. Whisk the egg whites until stiff but not dry.
7. Carefully fold in the egg whites and the chocolate drops, return the mixture to the freezer container and freeze.
8. 30 minutes before serving, remove from the freezer and place in the fridge.

Serves 6 *55 calories per portion*

Puddings (Cold)

There is nothing like a chilly choccy pudding to tickle your taste buds at the end of a meal. These are all quick to prepare so save some calories for them from your daily allowance.

CHOCCY CHESTNUT MOUSSE

275ml skimmed milk
3 level tbsp (45ml) cocoa
sweetener
175g chestnut purée
2tbsp (30ml) hot water
1 sachet (10g) gelatine
2 egg whites

1. Heat 150ml milk to boiling point.
2. Mix cocoa to a paste with some of the remaining milk.
3. Blend the hot milk with the cocoa and then place back in the pan and bring to the boil.

4. Remove from the heat and cool slightly.

5. Add sweetener to taste.

6. Place in a blender with the chestnut puree and the rest of the milk, and mix until smooth.

7. Dissolve the gelatine in the hot water and add to the blender. Mix again.

8. Place in a bowl and refrigerate until the mousse just starts to set.

9. Whisk the egg whites until stiff but not dry. Fold into the chocolate mixture.

10. Divide between 4 individual serving dishes and chill.

Serves 4 *165 calories per portion*

CHOCOLATE MINTY MERINGUES

25g Mint Matchmakers, broken into small pieces

100g mint choc ice cream

4 meringue nests

4tbsp (60ml) Cadbury's Chocolate Liqueur

chocolate, for decoration

1. Fold the broken Matchmakers into the ice cream.

2. Spoon a portion into each meringue nest.

3. Sprinkle with liqueur and decorate with a small amount of chocolate.

Serves 4 *205 calories per portion*

CHOCOLATE MOUSSE

1 carton (215g) Carnation Light unsweetened condensed semi-skimmed milk (or tin)
2 level tsp (10ml) powdered gelatine
4tbsp (60ml) water
1 sachet Ovaltine Options Choc-n-Orange or Choc-O-lait
mandarin segments to decorate

1. Chill the carton of Carnation Light overnight.
2. Sprinkle the gelatine on to 2tbsp (30ml) of cold water in a cup. Leave to soak for 5 minutes.
3. Stand the cup in a pan containing a little simmering water and leave until the gelatine is dissolved or microwave on Defrost for 30 seconds.

4. Mix the Ovaltine Options with 2tbsp (30ml) hot water to make a smooth paste.

5. Whip the Carnation Light until very frothy. Continue whipping while adding the dissolved gelatine and chocolate mixture.

6. Turn into a serving dish or 4 individual dishes and chill until set. Decorate with mandarin segments.

Serves 4 *80 calories per portion*

CHOCOLATE PEAR TRIFLE

3 trifle sponges
3 level tsps (15ml) reduced-sugar jam
425g can pears in juice
2tbsp (30ml) cherry brandy
225ml orange juice
275ml water
1 sachet (10g) gelatine
3 level tbsp (45ml) Hermesetas Sprinkle Sweet
3 level tbsp (45ml) custard powder
1 level tbsp (15ml) cocoa
425ml semi-skimmed milk
25g flaked almonds

Chock full of Taste!

1. Split the trifle sponges and fill with jam. Place in a glass bowl.
2. Drain the pears and reserve the juice. Mix 2tbsp (30ml) juice with the cherry brandy and sprinkle over the sponges.
3. Mix the remaining juice with the orange juice and make up to 1 pint (575ml) with water.
4. Dissolve the gelatine in the juice and add 1 level tbsp (15ml) Sprinkle Sweet. Pour over the sponges and chill until set.
5. Mix the custard powder and cocoa with a little milk until smooth.
6. Heat the remaining milk until almost boiling and then add to the custard mixture, stirring continuously. Return to the pan and bring to the boil while stirring. Simmer for 2 minutes.
7. Pour into a cool basin and add the remaining Sprinkle Sweet. Leave to cool, whisking lightly very frequently.
8. Pour over the jelly. Toast the almonds and sprinkle on top.

Serves 6 *180 calories per portion*

CHOCOLATE POTS WITH COINTREAU

2 eggs, size 3

2 level tbsp (30ml) cocoa

425ml skimmed milk

2tbsp (30ml) Cointreau

Hermesetas Sprinkle Sweet, to taste

orange peel

4 squirts of aerosol cream to decorate

1. Whisk the eggs with the cocoa powder in a bowl.
2. Heat the milk almost to boiling point and gradually add to the egg mixture stirring all the time.
3. Set the bowl over a pan of simmering water and cook stirring constantly until the mixture thickens.
4. Strain into ramekin dishes and stand in a deep roasting tin.
5. Pour hot water into the roasting tin to come halfway up the sides of the ramekins.
6. Cover with greaseproof paper and bake in the oven at 170°C, 325°F, Gas 3 for 25–30 minutes or until just set.
7. Allow to cool and serve decorated with a squirt of

Anchor Light aerosol cream and a thin strip of orange peel.

Serves 4 *155 calories per portion*

Puddings (Hot)

Centuries ago, chocolate was served hot as a rather bitter-tasting drink. The cocoa flavour develops a smoothness and richness when hot and, these days, you can add a sweet taste without too many extra calories by using a sugar substitute.

CHOCOLATE AND CHERRY STEAMED PUDDING

75g margarine
4 level tbsp (60ml) Hermesetas Sprinkle Sweet
2 eggs, size 2
150g self-raising flour
15g cocoa

$^{1}/_{2}$ level tsp (2.5ml) baking powder

4 tbsp (60ml) semi-skimmed milk

75g glacé cherries

1. Cream the margarine and Sprinkle Sweet together.
2. Lightly beat the eggs and then add to the creamed mixture a little at a time, beating well after each addition.
3. Sieve together the flour, cocoa and baking powder and then add to the mixture with the milk and cherries.
4. Turn into a greased basin and cover with greaseproof paper and foil. Steam for $1^{1}/_{2}$ hours. Serve with chocolate sauce (*see* recipe on page 201).

CHOCOLATE AND RAISIN RICE PUDDING

40g pudding rice

3 level tbsp (45ml) Hermesetas Sprinkle Sweet

50g raisins

2 level tsp (10ml) cocoa

575ml semi-skimmed milk

1. Place the rice, Sprinkle Sweet and raisins in an ovenproof dish.
2. Mix the cocoa with a little of the milk until smooth
3. Add the remaining milk and pour over the rice.
4. Bake at 150°C, 300°F, Gas 2 for about 2 hours. Stir after $1/2$ hour and again after 1 hour.

Serves 4 *150 calories per portion*

CHOCOLATE BAKED CUSTARD

100g fresh white breadcrumbs
1 pint (575ml) skimmed milk
3 level tbsp (45ml) cocoa
Hermesetas Sprinkle Sweet
1 egg, size 3, lightly beaten

1. Place the breadcrumbs in a 850ml ovenproof dish.
2. Blend 2tbsp (30ml) of the skimmed milk with the cocoa until smooth.
3. Gradually stir in the remaining milk and pour into a saucepan and bring to the boil.
4. Add Sprinkle Sweet to taste.

5. Pour the cocoa mixture over the egg, stirring all the time and then strain over the breadcrumbs.
6. Leave to stand for 20 minutes and then bake for 45–50 minutes at 180°C, 350°F, Gas 4.

Serves 4 *160 calories per portion*

CHOCOLATE FONDUE (Microwave recipe)
fresh fruit, cut into chunks or strips
100g plain chocolate drops
275ml Shape Single
150ml unsweetened orange juice

1. Arrange fruit 'dippers' on a plate and sprinkle with lemon juice.
2. Place the chocolate drops, Shape Single and orange juice in a 1-litre bowl and microwave on Medium for 10–12 minutes until the mixture blends together, stirring twice throughout the cooking time.
3. Serve immediately with cocktail sticks to spear fruit.

Serves 4 *300 calories per portion*

CHOCOLATE SAUCE

4 level tbsp (60ml) custard powder

2 level tbsp (30ml) cocoa

850ml semi-skimmed milk

3 level tbsp (45ml) Hermesetas Sprinkle Sweet

1. Mix the custard powder and cocoa with a little of the milk until smooth.
2. Heat the remaining milk until almost boiling.
3. Pour on to the custard powder, stirring all the time.
4. Return to the pan and bring to the boil, stirring continuously. Simmer for 2 minutes.
5. Remove from the heat and stir in the Sprinkle Sweet.

Serves 8 *75 calories per portion*

CHOCOLATE SEMOLINA

275ml semi-skimmed milk

2 level tbsp (15ml) semolina

25g chocolate hazelnut spread

Hermesetas Sprinkle Sweet to taste

1. Heat the milk in a small pan nearly to boiling point.
2. Add in the semolina and cook gently for 2 minutes stirring all the time.
3. Remove from the heat and stir in the chocolate hazelnut spread and Sprinkle Sweet before serving.

Serves 2–3 *About 200 calories per portion*

MINI CHOC PUD (Microwave recipe)

15g low-fat spread
3 tsp (15ml) plain flour
Hermesetas Sprinkle Sweet
65ml milk
25g plain chocolate drops
1 egg, size 3, separated
pinch of cream of tartar

1. Microwave the low-fat spread on High for 15 seconds.
2. Sift the flour into the low-fat spread, then add the sweetener and the milk.
3. Microwave on High for 1 minute or until thickened, stirring once.

4. Add the chocolate drops and stir until melted.

5. Beat the egg yolk into the chocolate mixture.

6. Whisk the egg white with the cream of tartar until it is stiff but not dry and fold carefully into the chocolate mixture.

7. Turn into a lightly greased dish and microwave on Defrost for 2 minutes. Serve immediately.

Serves 1 *360 calories per portion*

CHOCCY SANDWICHES AND NIBBLES

These are quick, tasty treats which need no cooking. Remember to eat them slowly, enjoying every mouthful.

- Sandwich of 2 slices wholemeal bread, 1 small sliced banana, 2 tsp (10ml) drinking chocolate. *250 calories*
- Sandwich of 2 slices slimmer's bread, toasted or plain, 25g Cadbury's Chocolate Spread. *165 calories*
- Toasted treat of 1 slice wholemeal toast, topped with orange slices and 1 squirt Anchor Light Chocolate Mousse. *200 calories*

- Open sandwich of 1 slice wholemeal bread, topped with 2 tsps (10ml) reduced-sugar strawberry jam, 1 squirt aerosol cream, 1 sliced fun-size Mars bar. *275 calories*
- Naughty nibble of 2 crispbreads topped with 2 tsp (10ml) reduced-sugar raspberry jam, 1 Cadbury's Wispa cut in two and crumbled up. *125 calories*

10

The Chocaholic's Food Diary

Keep a weekly food diary to help you stick to your diet. All you need is a notebook, divided into columns as shown overleaf. Keep it with you at all times so that you can make a note of your mood, where you were, and who you were with during each meal, snack or nibble. Once a week, analyse it yourself, using the ten pointers below.

If you feel that you have your chocoholic problem well and truly under control and don't need the diary any more, fine. However, if your weight creeps up again, or you find that your thoughts (and fingers!) are repeatedly straying towards chocolate, fill in a diary for a week, and you'll be able to nip problems in the bud before they get out of control.

POINTS TO CHECK

1. Note the time, place and mood you were in when you had difficulty in controlling choc-eating urges. Were you under pressure? Had you eaten enough during the day? Were others making your life difficult? Think about it.

2. Did you eat properly at breakfast time? If not, is there a way of making things easier — preparing your food the night before perhaps, or getting up a bit earlier? Maybe it is not as bad as it sounds and it would make tempers less frayed all round. I get up at 6.45am and enjoy a leisurely breakfast and read the papers before starting work at 8.30am. It is worth it, honestly.

3. Did you sit down and eat your meals in a proper, civilised atmosphere? If you snatched something at a

station or from a takeaway, chances are your brain didn't get a chance to register 'full' signals properly because you ate the food in such a rush. This could explain why you snacked again later in the day.

4. Is there a pattern to your snack-attacks? Does a particular person, place, TV programme trigger them? By recognising these patterns you are already half-way to curing the problem.

5. Are your meals really satisfying? If you have noted tummy rumblings throughout the day, it could be that you are not eating enough. Don't forget to pile on those 'free' vegetables and check that you are consuming everything you are allowed on your eating programme.

6. Are you exposing yourself to unnecessary temptation by not being prepared? Look for occasions when you went astray because you didn't have the right low-calorie snacks with you. Plan to set this right immediately. It takes only a few seconds to pop a

packet of low-fat crisps and some fruit into your bag or briefcase but it could prevent you from eating several bars of chocolate later on.

7. Do you need to shop more often? It's crazy to ruin your diet because you don't have the right foods in the larder. Check if there were times when you ate something unsuitable just because there was nothing better in the house. Vow to shop more intelligently next week, adding the things you need to your list.

8. Are you leaving gaps that are too long between meals? This can happen if you are not prepared. See above!

9. Did stress or a family upset make you 'comfort eat'? If so, forgive yourself and try to deal with similar problems in a different way next time. Don't forget that exercise is a great stress-beater.

10. Did you do exceptionally well? Congratulate yourself and give yourself a treat immediately. If it's a

choccy one, make sure it is within your daily calorie allowance and combine it with some other sensual pleasure like listening to music, or relaxing in the bath!

THE   CHOCAHOLIC'S

	Monday	Tuesday	Wednesday
Breakfast: Where? Who with Mood	Poached egg on toast At home, kitchen Children, Husband Irritable. Forced to eat grabbing mouthfuls family problems		
Lunch: Where? Who with Mood	Chicken sandwich packet of crisps Office, alone Cross with myself for eating crisps Work horrendous		
Supper Where? Who with Mood	Prawn tikka, boiled rice poppadam, half lager Indian restaurant Four mates Resisted nan bread/ fried rice; will have fruit at home		
Bedtime Where? Who with Mood	Ovaltine Options drink in bed Alone, husband watching TV Good. Feel positive		

FOOD   DIARY

Thursday	Friday	Saturday	Sunday

Calorie Guide to
Your Favourite Chocs

On the Chocaholic Diet, you are allowed a certain amount of chocolate. Choose it from this list. For your convenience, we have divided certain chocolate products into calorie-counted sections. These are fun-size (mostly under 100 calories), under 100 calories, 200, 250, and 300 calories.

There is also a list of chocolate biscuit products, cakes, individual chocolates, chocolate liqueurs, specialist products and even choc-erotica. Remember, watch those calories and divide larger treats up into smaller daily portions if you prefer. Alternatively, you can save your chocolate allowance for one or two nights to nibble at it. It is better to buy your allowance daily to avoid any temptation.

FUN SIZE

	Calories
Cadbury's	
Buttons	75
Crunchie	80
Dairy Milk	80
Double Decker	85
Fudge	60
Wispa	80
Mars	
Bounty miniature	39
Maltesers	106
Mars	90
Milky Way	76
Snickers	162
Nestlé	
Aero	58

Lion Bar	78
Smarties	68

UNDER 100 CALORIES
Cadbury's
Flake (treat size)	80

Kinder
Chocolate Mini Bar	65

Nestlé
Milky Bar	69
Smarties (mini)	68

UNDER 150 CALORIES
Boots
Shapers Bars	100

Cadbury's
Chomp	120
Crunchie (small)	130
Curly Wurly	115

Fudge	120
Ruffle	125
Taz	85
Twirl (finger)	115
Wildlife Bar	115

Kinder

| Surprise Egg | 110 |

Mars

| Milky Way (single) | 118 |
| Twix Tea Break | 144 |

Nestlé

| Kit Kat (2 fingers) | 108 |
| Drifter (finger) | 135 |

Marks and Spencer

| Walnut Whip | 120 |

UNDER 200 CALORIES
Cadbury's

| Buttons (standard) | 175 |
| Creme Egg | 175 |

Crunchie (standard)	195
Flake	180
Wispa (snack)	125

Fry's

Chocolate Cream	215
Peppermint Cream	215
Turkish Delight	175

Marks and Spencer

Amaretto Bar	203
Chunky Caramel Bar	236

Mars

Mars (snack size)	190
Revels (small)	175

Nestlé

Aero (chunky)	191
Dairy Crunch	160
Lion Bar	247
Milky Bar	175
Milky Bar Buttons	180
Caramac (small)	164
Smarties (tube)	170
Walnut Whip, Vanilla	167

UNDER 250 CALORIES
Cadbury's

Caramel	240
Double Decker	230
Fruit & Nut (chunky)	240
Picnic	230
Spira (2 pieces)	210

Mars

Galaxy	250
m&ms (standard)	219
Milky Way (twin)	236
Topic	234

Nestlé

Kit Kat (4 finger)	247
Milky Bar (chunky)	203
Toffee Crisp	238

UNDER 300 CALORIES
Cadbury's

Bournville	250
Dairy Milk	255
Whole Nut	265

Mars

Bounty (twin)	276
Maltesers	289
Mars (standard)	294

Nestlé

Munchies	261
Rolo (medium)	270

INDIVIDUAL SWEETS

Nestlé

After Eight Mint	35

Elizabeth Shaw

After Dinner Mint	40
Harvey's Bristol Cream Truffle	60
Irish Cream Truffle	60
Mint Crisp or Orange Crisp	28

Ferrero Rocher

Per choc	75
Mon Cheri	38

Marks and Spencer

After Dinner Mint	32
Chocolate Eclair Sweet	33
Extremely Chocolate Caramel	37

Thorntons

Chocolate Brazil	66
Coconut Paradise	60
Coffee Cream	55

CHOC-EROTICA

Spencer and Fleetwood

Naughty Bits selection
(calories per individual chocolate):

Drunken Bum	59
Nipple	81
Belgian Chocolate Willie	540
(90g solid chocolate)	
Boob	540
(90g solid chocolate)	
Cream Filled Willie (100g)	684

CHOCOLATE BISCUITS

(Per Biscuit)

ASDA

Choc Chip Cookie	56
Jaffa Cake	45
Milk Chocolate Digestive	84
Milk Chocolate Nice	61

Burton's

Chocolate Digestive	78
Jaffa Cake	46
Milk Chocolate Royal Tea	54
Wagon Wheel	164

Cadbury's

Chocolate Finger	29
Snack Sandwich	140

Co-Op

Choc Chip Cookie	48
Choc Chip Shortbread	98
Milk Choc Country Crunch	82
Milk Choc Orange Wafer	44

Crawfords

Choc Chip Oatie	37
Milk Chocolate Finger	37
Plain Chocwheat	65

Jacob's

Chocolate Chip Shortbread	88
Gems Chocolate	60
Ginger and Choc Chip	84
Triple Chocolate Crumble	93
Vitelinea Crispy Chocolate Biscuit	14

Marks and Spencer

Chocolate Chip Cookie	58
Jaffa Cake	47
Milk Chocolate Digestive	88
Milk Chocolate Viennese Swirl	88
Reduced Fat Milk Chocolate Digestive	77

McVitie's

Go Ahead Plain Chocolate Chocolini	55
Chocolate Hob Nob Cream	73
Jaffa Cake	48
Milk Chocolate Ginger Nut	70

Mini Jaffa Cake	26
Munchmallow	76

Prewett's
Chocolate Flapjack	142
Giant Double Chocolate Chip	249

Quaker
Chocolate Chip Harvest Chewy Bar	101
Chocolate Orange Chip	98

Sainsbury's
American Style Choco Chip Cookie	90
Choc and Nut Cookie	58
Chocolate Chip Digestive	70
Jaffa Cake	48
Milk Chocolate Digestive Finger	46

Tesco
Chocolate Chip Cereal Bar	125
25% Less Fat Milk Chocolate Digestive	74

Walkers
Hazelnut and Chocolate Chip	88

Orange and Chocolate Chip	81
Plain Chocolate Ginger Royal	64
Chocolate Chip Shortbread	103

Weight Watchers

Real Chocolate Chip Cookie	98

CHOCOLATE BREAKFAST CEREALS

(28g portion)

Co-Op

Chop Chip Muesli	114
Choco Dinosaurs	108
Chocolate and Strawberry Crisp	130
Chocolate Cornflakes	104

Kellog's

Choco Corn Flakes	108
Choco Krispies	108

Marks and Spencer

Chocolate Crunch	126

Nestlé

Nesquick Cereal   108

Safeway

Choc Flakes   108
Chocolate and Strawberry Crunch   132
Coco Crunchies   107

Sainsbury's

Choco Hoops   122
Coco Snaps   108

Somerfield

Cocoa Rice   106

Sunblest

Swiss Style Chocolate Flavour Cornflakes   109

Tesco

Choco Crunchies   119
Cocoa Cornflakes   106
Cocoa Puffs   109

Waitrose

Choc and Hazelnut Crunch	139
Chocolate, Toffee and Banana Crunch	123

CHOCOLATE CAKES

(Per cake unless otherwise stated)

ASDA

Chocolate Coated Caramel Cake Bar	137
Chocolate Mini Roll with Vanilla	96
Real Milk Chocolate Rice Crisp Cake	115
Chocolate Eclair (66g)	255
Chocolate Sponge	230
Chocolate Fudge Cake (60g slice)	250
Chocolate Swiss Roll (28g slice)	112

Cadbury's

Chocolate Flake Cake	242
Chocolate Mini Roll	112
Milk Chocolate Cake Bar	115

Entemann's

Chocolate Fudge Brownie, 28g slice	87

Double Chocolate Muffin	153
Chocolate Orange Cake, 28g slice	113
Mississipi Mud Cake, 28g slice	128

Fry's

| Turkish Delight Cake | 91 |

Lyons

Chocolate Cup Cake	132
Chocolate Swiss Roll	115
Chocolate Trifle Sponge	65

Marks and Spencer

Fudge Brownie	236
Chocolate Éclair	155
Choux Bun	247

McVitie's

Chocolate Dream Cake Bar	143
Double Chocolate Cake Bar	93
Jaffa Cake Bar	129

Mr Kipling

| Black Forest Slice | 165 |

Chocolate Chip Cake Bar	146
Chocolate Fudge Brownie Cake Bar	143
Double Chocolate Cake Bite	43
Mini Chocolate Sponge	163

Waitrose

Chocolate Buttercream Log (28g slice)	106
Chocolate Chip Cake (28g slice)	115
Coconut Chocolae Fudge Cake	125

DRINKS

Alcoholic: (25ml pub measure)

Cadbury's Chocolate Cream Liqueur	75
Sainsbury's White Chocolate and Hazelnut Cream Liqueur	86

BEVERAGES

Cadbury's

Per sachet:

Bournville Plain Chocolate Break	118
Chocolate Break	118

Highlights, all flavours	40

Per 28g dry powder:

Cocoa	91
Drinking Chocolate	104

Co-Op
Per 28g dry powder:

Drinking Chocolate	107
Instant Chocolate Drink	115

Horlicks
Per 28g dry powder:

Low Fat Instant Chocolate Malt	108
Low Fat Instant Hot Chocolate	109

Per sachet:

Maltissimo Milk Chocolat, Mocha, or Tiramisu	65

Kraft Jacobs Suchard
Per sachet:

Terry's Chocolate Orange drink	70
Toblerone drink	70

Nestlé

Per sachet:

Chococino	87
Chococino Light	39
Nescafe au Chocolat	70

Options

Per sachet:

Choc and Ginger, Choc and Mint, etc	39
Ultimate Chocolate Indulgence	76
White Chocolate	55

Suchard

Per Sachet:

Suchard Hot Chocolate Drink	91

CHOCOLATE ICE CREAM

ASDA

Choc Fudge Italian Ice cream Cone	208
Choc Ice Dark	137
Choc Ice Light	138
Chocolate Classic	183

Give Me Choc Lolly Milk Choc	179
Mighty Chocolate Bar	200

Ben and Jerry's
Per 28g scoop:

Chocolate Chip Cookie Dough	77
Chocolate Fudge Brownie	73
Chunky Monkey	79

Cadbury's

Ice Cream Chocolates, each	65
Crunchie	183

Co-Op

Choc and Nut Ice Cream Cone	307
Choc Ice Dark	102
Choc Ice Light	117
Choc Ice Neopolitan	123

Häagen-Dazs
Per 28g scoop

Belgian Chocolate	78
Chocolate Choc Chip	77

Lyons Maid

Chocolate Mousse	83
Classico Dark or Light Choc Ice	184
King Cone Mint Chocolate Chip	185

Marks and Spencer

Per 28g scoop:

Double Chocolate Crunch	86
Homestyle Chocolate	73
Mint Chocolate	79

Individual items:

Belgian Milk Chocolate Bar	321
Milk Choc Ice	175

Mars

Bounty Stick	299
Galaxy Milk	299
Mars or Mars Dark	210
Snickers	230
Twix	231
Pick 'n' Mix Minis, Mars, Milky Way, etc.	60

Nestlé

Aero	218
Kit Kat	218
Lion Bar	265
Rolo	163

Sainsbury's

Belgian Chocolate Extravaganza Bar	228

Per 28g scoop:

Jaffa Chocolate Orange	56
Mint Chocolate	64
Chocoholic Cherry Ecstasy	78

Wall's

Chunky Choc Bar	165
Magnum Orange Chocolate	295
Mini Milk Chocolate	35

Per 28g scoop:

Gino Ginelli Choc Choc Chip	60
Carte d'Or Chocolate	70

Weight Watchers
Per 28g scoop:
Chocolate Swirl   28

ALL OF THESE ARE LESS THAN 150 CALS

Sachet of Low Calorie chocolate
                              40 (1.4g fat)
Low-fat chocolate Mousse, small pot
                              85 (2.4g fat)
5 tbsp Coco Pops with skimmed milk
                              100 (0.5g fat)
Weight Watchers from Heinz Chocolate Tiramisu
                              141 (2.9g fat)
Sara Lee Mini Chocolate Chip Cheesecake Bite
                              100 (5.3g fat)
Marks and Spencer Chocolate and Mint Sundae
                              113 (3.8g fat)

Counselling Groups and Useful Contacts

If you feel that you need expert help to control your chocoholism, don't hesitate to seek it. In the first instance, you should consult your GP. The contacts below are all recommended, or write to me at the address below.

Promis Counselling Centre, London and Kent
Tel: 0207 581 8222
FREE 24-hour helpline: 0800 374 318
They offer one to one counselling or residential treatment for all addictive illnesses and GP referrals are possible.

Diabetes UK
PO Box 400
Swindon SN2 8LA
Tel: 0207 323 1531
Caroline: 0207 636 6112
They give information and help for diabetics and their families. If you suspect that you are diabetic, you must check with your doctor immediately. Many sufferers go undiagnosed for years. Symptoms are: thirst, tiredness, frequent passing of water.

National Centre for Eating Disorders
54 New Road
Esher
Surrey KT10 9NU
Tel: 01327 469493
This is a network of fully trained counsellors, offering one to one personal treatment plus phone counselling. The Centre was started by Deanne Jade, a psychologist and leading expert on eating and weight problems. In some cases, the Centre may be able to help you obtain treatment via your GP.

Overeaters Anonymous   07000 784 985

If you would like to write to me, my address is:
Sally Ann Voak
PO Box 618
Coulsdon
Surrey CR5 1RU